CURRENT AND FUTURE TRENDS
IN COMMUNITY PSYCHOLOGY

CURRENT AND FUTURE TRENDS IN COMMUNITY PSYCHOLOGY

Edited by

Stuart E. Golann, Ph.D.
Professor of Psychology
University of Massachusetts
Amherst

Jeffrey Baker
Department of Psychology
University of Massachusetts
Amherst

Human Sciences Press

A division of Behavioral Publications, Inc.
New York

Library of Congress Catalog Number 74-8507

ISBN: 0-87705-146-1

HUMAN SCIENCES PRESS
72 Fifth Avenue
New York, New York 10011

Printed in the United States of America
56789 987654321

Library of Congress Cataloging in Publication Data

Golann, Stuart E
    Current and future trends in community psychology.

    Papers originally presented as a series of lectures presented
at the University of Massachusetts, Amherst, Feb. -May, 1973.
    Bibliography: p.
    1. Community psychology—Addresses, essays, lectures.
I. Baker, Jeffrey, 1943-   joint author.   II.   Title.
[DNLM: 1. Community mental health services.
2.   Psychology, Social. WM30 G616c]
RC455.G58   362.2   74-8507

CONTRIBUTORS

Jack M. Chinsky
Associate Professor of Psychology, University of Connecticut

Ira Iscoe
Professor of Psychology and Education, and Director, Graduate Training in Community Mental Health, The University of Texas at Austin

J. Robert Newbrough
Professor of Psychology, and Coordinator, Center for Community Studies, George Peabody College

Gershen Rosenblum
Region V Mental Health Administrator, Department of Mental Health, Commonwealth of Massachusetts

Edison J. Trickett
Assistant Professor, Department of Psychology; and Institution for Social and Policy Studies, Yale University

CONTENTS

Introduction   1

1. Community Psychology, 1973: With a
   View Backward and Forward   13
   J. R. Newbrough

2. Collaborative Interventions in Community
   Mental Health: A Personal Perspective   41
   Jack M. Chinsky

3. Community Psychology and Mental Health
   Administration: From the Frying Pan
   Into the Fire   83
   Gershen Rosenblum

4. The Educating of a Community Psychologist   123
   Edison J. Trickett

5. Becoming a Community Psychologist   181
   Ira Iscoe

Index   223

ACKNOWLEDGMENT

We would like to express our appreciation to Ms. Sara Ives, typesetter and proofreader, and Ms. Diana Scriver, indexer.

INTRODUCTION

> Although clinical psy-
> chology is closely related to
> medicine, it is quite as close-
> ly related to sociology and to
> pedagogy. The school room, the
> juvenile court, and the streets
> are a larger laboratory of psy-
> chology. An abundance of ma-
> terial for scientific study
> fails to be utilized because
> the interests of psychologists
> are elsewhere engaged . . .
> (Witmer, 1907).

Although concepts of community psychology are not new, the term "community
psychology" first emerged at the Swampscott Conference in May, 1965. Convened
for a conference on the education of psychologists in community mental health,
the participants with unusual consensus
moved toward a conception of community
psychology as a _field_, community mental
health as one _area of interest_ in this
field, and clinical psychology as one
specialty area relevant to community mental health. Swampscott marked the beginning of an enlarged system of constructs

1

and of greater aspirations for psychology. In fact, although nobody called it
that, it was sort of a "Psych Lib" meeting with the consciousness raising and
personal exhilaration of such experiences.
For example, the group notes included several statements like the following one:

> There rapidly emerged a widely
> shared and strongly expressed group
> recognition that the participants
> had come to the Conference not mere-
> ly because of a concrete interest
> in the CMH movement but perhaps more
> importantly because of a more gener-
> al concern for the need to expand
> our professional area of inquiry and
> action beyond the traditional mold.
> It was suggested that a tentative
> label for the direction of the ex-
> pansion be "Community Psychology."
> Movement in this direction is dic-
> tated by our own intrinsic profes-
> sional judgment and feelings of com-
> petence and not by such extrinsic
> factors as Federal program guide-
> lines or the availability of ear-
> marked monies.

> "Community Psychology" was de-
> scribed as an interest in general
> psychological processes that link
> conceptually the societal level and
> individual behavior, the clarifica-
> tion of such linkage serving as a
> rational basis for action programs
> for optimizing human functioning.
> Included in the sphere of interest
> would be, for example, studies of
> planned change, involvement of indi-
> viduals and groups in active mas-

tery of the environment, psychological ecology, effects of social action, normal human development in
the broad sense, group tension-sol-
ving strategems, etc.

Reports of this conference (Bennett,
1965; Bennett, Anderson, Cooper, Hassol,
Klein, & Rosenblum, 1966) became working
drafts of a constitution of a new area of
psychology, eager to be free of the ideo-
logical constraints of illness-centered
explanations of human events, and aspir-
ing to understand and respond to persons
in their varied individual and social
contexts.

Several years have elapsed since and
among notable landmarks are: the formation of a Division of Community Psychology
within the American Psychological Association; the publication of the Community
Mental Health Journal, now in its eighth
year; the beginning of two new journals,
the American Journal of Community Psychology and the Journal of Community Psychology in 1973; and in the interim a rapidly increasing number of monographs, books,
and other publications relevant to community psychology or mental health (see
Cowen, 1973). Graduate training programs
included increasing content and practice
relevant to community psychology and mental health and individual psychologists
have increasingly been involved in new
service and research roles. All of these
attest to the continued existence and probable growth of community psychology and
mental health.

Scribner (1970), however, asks, "What is community psychology made of?" and points out how difficult it is to answer the question adequately. "Some answers characterize the motivations and value systems of individuals attracted to the field ...; some point to new work settings ...; some emphasize the employment of new skills and techniques ...; still others speak of a common point of view toward the practical uses of psychological knowledge and methodology." Scribner concludes that community psychology represents the bringing together of various psychologists concerned with the broad questions of man in society and that the question "What is community psychology?" should really be "Who are these psychologists? What if anything do they have in common?"

To the organizers of the series of lectures reported in this book, it seemed that the best way to answer these and other questions about the content and directions of community psychology was to ask a group of active community psychologists what they are doing. It is an unfortunate fact that most subsequent attempts to define community psychology have not recaptured the adventure of the Swampscott meeting. To the contrary, they often become frustrating semantic exercises with words and slogans failing to convey the excitements and frustrations of ongoing research and practice.

The lecture series, which ran from February to May, 1973, on the campus of the University of Massachusetts, Amherst, was therefore suggested not to define

community psychology in the traditional
sense, but to define it five times over,
each time in a very personal sense. Each
of the participants was asked to do the
same thing: "As a general suggestion
please try to develop a personal analysis of where community psychology has
been during the last decade and where you
see it heading during the coming decade.
Emphasize your own development of interest in community psychology and illustrate the meaning community psychology
has for you by presenting in some detail
an example of your recent activities."
Each participant, then, was asked to show
how he translates belief into action, to
be something of an historian-futurist,
but mostly to present himself and his research or applied work as a definition of
community psychology in action. The participants were asked to candidly describe
some aspects of their current work and to
attempt to share their experiences and
aspirations with us. Knowing where they
have been and which way they are going
can provide a perspective on where community psychology has been and where it
is going.

Major involvement in community psychology was the basic criterion used to
select the participants and fortunately
the five persons invited all accepted.
They also were chosen to represent different generations of community psychologists, with Iscoe, Newbrough, and Rosenblum having had a longer involvement in
psychology than Chinsky and Trickett.

The series was opened by Robert Newbrough. In his presentation he describes

the exploration and synthesis which have
brought him to his current conceptions of
community and psychology. These are
realized in his present research program
monitoring community events and individual
mood. His paper illustrates the uses of
multidisciplinary collaboration in community growth and future planning; attacks
the issue of change agentry that has con-
fused community psychology for a decade;
sharpens the picture of the community
psychologist as an integrated scientist-
professional; and raises questions, in-
escapable in a community psychology which
has grown up, of the potential uses and
abuses of technology and its enormous information yield to enhance or deplete the
quality of life in the community.

Newbrough's paper shows his long-
standing and wide interest in psychological theory. Most often he tries to put
theory to work; recently he has done research using psychophysical methods and
sociological theory to define and measure
deviant behavior. After several years at
the NIMH Mental Health Study Center, Newbrough moved to George Peabody College
where he now fills three roles: Professor of Psychology; Coordinator of Community Psychology Training; and Coordinator,
Center for Community Studies.

Jack Chinsky was next, describing
the beginnings of his involvement in community psychology with Emory Cowen and
Julian Rappaport while a graduate student
at Rochester during the social turbulence
of the 1960's. At the University of Connecticut since, Chinsky has concentrated
on the implementation and evaluation of

diverse community projects, using what he
terms the "collaborative intervention design" to maximize program impact for all
concerned. Chinsky's report illustrates
well the demandingness of multivariate,
service-oriented research. Just a few of
the necessary ingredients for successful
community interventions, clearly evidenced
in Chinsky's descriptions, are patience,
interpersonal skills, organizational planning ability, a willingness to make research open-ended, and perhaps above all
a capacity for energetic and creative involvement. Chinsky demonstrates that
meaningful research can be applied to social problems, with educational and community benefits. His predictions for community psychology's future are also provocative.

       The third speaker to come to the Uni-
versity of Massachusetts was Gershen Rosenblum. Rosenblum, among the five, is the
most involved in community mental health
services and administration. In 1967,
following seven years as Chief Psychologist at the South Shore Mental Health
Center (one of the first community-oriented
clinics and the first to have a community
training program for psychologists), Rosenblum became the Mental Health Administrator for Region V in the Massachusetts Department of Mental Health. He describes
in his paper how he came to the job and
the problems he has faced since. He has
been in an excellent position to describe
the full scope of challenges confronted
by psychologists active in the community.
He candidly describes the multifaceted
role of a mental health administrator--
drawing a detailed picture of what it

means, essentially, to be a community resource. The preventive emphasis, he
points out, is contributing to an evolution away from mental health services to
human services.

Ed Trickett became interested in community psychology through his work at Ohio
State University with James Kelly. In
"The Education of a Community Psychologist," he describes the path he took leading to his present position at Yale University where he has worked at the Psycho-
Educational Clinic and now is an Assistant Professor of Psychology and a member
of the Institution for Social and Policy
Studies. In his paper, Trickett shares
his efforts to develop an empirical research base in the study of person-setting
interaction and the assessment of settings
in and of themselves. His theoretical
orientation is that of ecological analogy
from field biology for analyzing social
environments; this he concretizes with
examples from his work doing assessment
of and consultation in high school settings. Trickett saved for last his concerns about the university as a setting
for the development of community psychology, weighing issues seldom explored
with the specificity he gives them.

The final speaker was Ira Iscoe, who
of the five speakers has been the most
involved in grass-roots community program development activities. He has been
working in the same community for 22 years
where he has become an expert in practical
politics of program survival and developed
long-standing allegiances within groups
which often are in conflict with each

other. In his unique, humorous but serious way, he describes in his paper how his
boyhood in Montreal, Canada, prepared him
for such activities. Iscoe then moves on
to discuss the pragmatics of service development, delivery, and evaluation, and
departures for community training which
are in his view inevitable (at the University of Texas, he has recently established a community mental health program outside the clinical area). Iscoe
touches all the issues, speaking more
experientially than theoretically. A
particularly useful theme running through
his presentation is that of the necessity
to explode the binds commonly imposed upon (and played into by) community psycho-
logists--most notably what Iscoe calls
"the promise to walk on water." His paper, like those that came before, is the
personal document of one who creates new
traditions in psychology.

          A decade ago, in the years just be-
fore and after the Swampscott meeting,
the field of psychology stood between established powerfulness and regulated
powerlessness. It was difficult to know
then if interest in community psychology
was the expression of a profession's conflict over further acquisition as against
further sharing of influence together
with an uncertainty about how to proceed
straightforwardly in either direction.
The emphases at the Swampscott Conference in 1965 were commitment to planned
social change; preventive interventions;
the furthering of normal development;
professional-community collaboration;
professional participation in community

affairs and a more intimate objectification; consultation to community institutions; interdisciplinary communication and collaboration in the sciences; development of interdisciplinary professional education; and development of innovative research methodologies appropriate to the study of complex systems.

In the work of five community psychologists in 1973, we see these same principles perpetuated and strengthened. If the participants are representative, then it appears that under the rubric of community psychology a large group of psychologists have freely defined "their psychology." The emphases in the talks delivered at the 1973 Symposium Series were, in particular, an attention to persons in settings, but more especially a sense of community as an entity man creates and depends upon for emotional and material support; a concern with conscious but flexible community planning to enhance human potentials and the quality of private and community living; and, most notably, the demystification of scientific research--that is, an insistence on grounded theory, and the reintegration of research into energetic, self-involving service and practice outside the laboratory.

REFERENCES

Bennett, C. C. Community psychology: Impressions of the Boston conference on the education of psychologists for community mental health. _American Psychologist_, 1965, _20_, 832-835.

Bennett, C. C., Anderson, L. S., Cooper, S., Hassol, L., Klein, D. C., & Rosenblum C. (Eds.) Community psychology: A report of the Boston conference on the education of psychologists for community mental health. Boston: Boston University Press, 1966.

Cowen, E. L. Social and community interventions. In P. H. Mussen & M. R. Rosenzweig (Eds.) Annual review of psychology, Volume 24. Palo Alto: Annual Reviews, Inc., 1973.

Scribner, S. What is community psychology made of? In P. E. Cook (Ed.) Community psychology and community mental health. San Francisco: Holden-Day, 1970. Pp. 13-20.

Witmer, L. Clinical psychology. Psychological Clinic, 1907, 1, 1-9.

1. COMMUNITY PSYCHOLOGY, 1973: WITH A VIEW BACKWARD AND FORWARD

J. R. Newbrough

In viewing the history of community psychology, I saw three bibliographies that stand as important landmarks leading to the development of the specialty area:

1. U. S. Public Health Service. Evaluation in mental health. Washington, D. C.: U. S. Government Printing Office, 1955.

2. Massachusetts General Hospital and Harvard Medical School. Community mental health and social psychiatry: A reference guide. Cambridge, Mass.: Harvard University Press, 1963.

3. Golann, S. Coordinate index reference to community mental health. New York: Behavioral Publications, 1969.

These were landmarks in community mental health where the concern primarily was with service delivery and where there was a great deal of interest in the evaluation of programs. The movement was advanced by the 1963 Community Mental Health Cen-

ters Act (PL-88-164) that led to a great
deal of public money being invested to
change the incidence of severe mental disorder.   The underlying approach was a
general public health model that, in the
long run, was directed toward preventing
mental disorder.   The event that cata-
lyzed the development of community psychology was the 1965 Swampscott Conference (Bennett et al., 1966) held for the
purpose of discussing how to train psychologists for community mental health.   The
fortuitous outcome of that conference was
an assertion that community psychology
was something more than community mental
health.   That marked the beginning of what
we are now calling community psychology.

ROOTS IN PSYCHOLOGY

While community psychology has very
strong roots in the history of psychology,
it does not seem to be merely another area
of applied psychology, defined by the area
of application.   I see community psychology as a molar psychology in the Lewinian
tradition (Newbrough, 1972).   Woodworth
introduced the organism between the S and
the R.   I propose an E that goes in between the R and the S; it stands for environment.   Community psychology then can
be said to take up where action research
left off (Sanford, 1970).

Another, and equally important, historical tradition comes from the perception research by Ames and Ittleson in
transactional functionalism (Allport,
1955; Cantril, 1960).   Community psychology, it would seem, tries to confront a

somewhat broader range of phenomena than
psychology has typically been concerned
with; namely, phenomena bounded on the
one end by existential and personal perceptions, and on the other end by global,
aggregated phenomena called the community.

There is an implication in the community psychology area for a new method in
science. The action research background,
practiced by Kurt Lewin, gives us a paradigm of the person in his setting as the
unit of analysis. I began this line of
thought in 1959 while trying to understand
what brought people to a mental health
center for treatment. I had tried several unsuccessful approaches to the analysis of the presenting problem and was at
a dead-end conceptually (Newbrough, 1965).
After I had moved to the Washington, D.C.,
area, I had dinner with a friend, Richard
B. Royce. It turned out that Royce had
training in language analysis and introduced me to Charles Morris (1946) and to
Arthur F. Bentley. He suggested that my
colleagues and I try a linguistic analysis of the presenting problem using Morris' modes of discourse categories. I
became very interested in the use of language as a way of describing behavior,
and more specifically, for understanding
the describer. I found myself regularly
coming across John Dewey's ideas of
functionalism and transactionalism. The
discussion of transactional-functional-
ism in Allport (1955) showed the Dewey
influence on Ames and Ittleson. Ames
struggled several years, recording his
thoughts in a personal journal (Cantril,
1960), to understand the relativity theory
view of the perceiver bringing percepts

to illusory stimuli and ways in which the
person learned this. Transaction was a
situation-specific event denoting a process of contact between persons and their
environment. I soon found myself reading
the original source on transactionalism,
Knowing and the Known (Dewey & Bentley,
1949). This has served as a conceptual
anchor point for me and has allowed me to
trace the Dewey influence into sociology
through Mead, Park, and Faris into philosophy (linguistics) via Charles Morris.

Dewey and Bentley (1949) used a frame
of reference that made real sense to me.
They postulated a three-way view of causality. There are theories which attri-
bute causality to the organism, called
self-actional. There are theories which
posit multiple causes which chain. These
are interactional; the interest here is
in the relationships between links in the
chain. The third type of theory is called
transactional; the approach here is that
phenomena have to be understood in their
contexts at a particular point in time
and are a product of the contemporary process and exchange. Reading this I had an
insight. I thought that this might be a
time of history similar to the hundred
years after the discoveries of Copernicus.
That period was one of conflict between
paradigms or frames of reference. We can
say the same about our own time. Social
conflict operates between people, some of
whom are seeing a certain kind of reality
and others who are seeing a different kind
of reality in the same process. In attempting to visualize transaction in a
behavioral frame of reference, I went to
human ecology because of the centrality

of the view of organism in its environments. This has been most helpful in giving me a context in which to consider process and transaction. Since then I have discovered general systems theory (von Bertalanffy, 1965) and reread Gestalt theory. For those interested in general systems theory, it would be profitable to go back and read some of the early Gestalt writers. I was startled to find Gestalt Theory to be our first approach to a kind of systems theory.

This intellectual odyssey also had added to it an interest in Arthur F. Bentley. I was curious who this man was who coauthored Dewey's last book. Arthur F. Bentley was a journalist for the Chicago Herald Tribune. He spent most of his life in Bloomington, Indiana, next to the University of Indiana. Bentley was a philosopher by avocation and wrote a number of philosophical articles. He crossed swords with many people, including J. R. Kantor, and was apparently instrumental in influencing Kantor's theory of interbehavioral psychology. He helped Dewey sort out the notion of transactionalism. Bentley wrote two very interesting articles, one called "The Human Skin: Philosophy's Last Line of Defense" (Bentley, 1941) where he argued that it is very difficult to limit phenomena as being either inside or outside the person. He published an article in 1950 in Science entitled "Kennetic Inquiry," in which he took on the issue of what behavioral relativity theory methodology would look like. He described a scientific approach which I call the "postulated observation of the environed organism." He thought

that one cannot understand except through
one's postulates or paradigms, but that
one should not try to understand only
through them. He must also try to get
information on the behavior in several
ways and see if he can find out what his
postulates are. One way is to observe
behavior in its environmental context.

Here was the stated need in science
to study both the observer and the observed. In a simplistic way, research
is a matter of positioning oneself in relationship to a phenomenon or a series of
phenomena and observing them in a certain
fashion. It should also include positioning others to observe you and to observe
the behavior (not unlike program evaluation nowadays). This is similar to what
Webb et al. (1966) and Denzin (1970) have
called the triangulation approach in research methods. They suggest that one
should measure phenomena in at least three
different ways so that one can triangulate
phenomena to see whether there is something that is reliable and replicable
under more than one condition.

This illustrates that community psychology has a proper and viable tradition
in psychology. It is a functionalistic
holism that continues the Lewinian tradition in a broader way.

ROOTS IN SOCIAL PSYCHOLOGY
AND SOCIAL CHANGE

Contemporary community psychology
contains two major lines of thought. One

is the extention of community mental health
psychology, which is a clinical psychology
taken into the community. The other is a
view called "social policy oriented work."
This involves organizational and systemic
concerns where the emphasis is on the environment and its change rather than on
the person and personal change. Those are
different paradigms; there are tensions
between them in the field. There is a
great deal of interest in new social pro-
gramming, social problem research, and a
major emphasis on program evaluation (see
Levin, 1970).

At the same time, the country is being substantially affected by the New
Federalism policies of President Nixon.
It had been experiencing a shift, during
the 50's and 60's, from an industrial to
a postindustrial mode. This means a
change from concern with production and
a production economy to a consumption economy where the purpose for life does not
have to be producing things, but rather
doing something with them for some other
purpose (Michael, 1962). That confronts
one with the issue of the purpose of living.

Social change, historically, has pi-
voted around a shift in power. Much of
social change has followed wars. Power
has shifted from nation to nation, with
the rise and decline of each nation's fate
generally viewed as a matter of dominance
and submission. Dominance was a Darwinism
evolutionary principle to justify the historical process as a matter of "nature"
whereby the best was selected. Hofstadter
(1970) describes social Darwinism as hav-

ing been superceded. There are some new
writings about an alternative (or win-win)
solution to conflicts for power and resources. Harvey Wheeler in Democracy in
a Revolutionary Era (1968) argued that
nations are in a state of connectedness
where wars, particularly for the purpose
of dominance, will become decreasingly
possible. Revel (1971), in Without Marx
or Jesus, suggested that there are five
streams of change going on simultaneously
in this country. New forms of power are
developing, and there seems to be a general diffusion of power. Some think that
it will probably lead to a voluntary society (Bauer, 1960; Schindler-Rainman &
Lippitt, 1971). The matter of power and
its diffusion into a voluntary society
would seem to me to be one of the great
challenges of community psychology.

These perspectives on social change
bring to the forefront the basic philosophical issue of community: the relationships of man to the group in getting
his needs met. Rousseau (1913) has postulated the relationship as conflictual,
with the needs of one or the other being
met. Rawls (1972) has suggested that
this relationship can be repostulated as
one being capable of mutual need-meeting.
Engineering uses the concept "synergy" to
describe two forces being brought together
to yield more energy. Thomas Gordon (1970)
describes win-win philosophies in child
rearing. Harris (1973) allows the self
to be OK and others to be OK at the same
time. The basic philosophy of community
is changing. Community forms can be expected to change. Community psychology
should be concerned with the impacts of

change and focus on the growth and development of citizens. The theory and practice of community psychology will involve design and planning as much as adaptive reactions to already extant forms.

THEORY OF COMMUNITY

Reiff (1970) and Levin (1970) feel that it is the responsibility of the community psychologist to work for shifts of political power. Social advocacy is a way of furthering this. My own interest in social philosophy is toward the question "What is community?" Max Weber (1966) suggested that the major community function is a market place. This is an historical view that people cannot meet all their basic needs alone. In order to meet those needs, they must produce a surplus of goods for trading in order to get the range of things necessary to support their own lives. So long as there is a fairly low-energy exchange system, human life stays rather close to the means of production and all aspects of social life stay in closer touch with each other. When one gets into a society like ours (very highly differentiated and using lots of energy) the city becomes a support for the market place. The market place is controlled by interests which are separated from the people who live and work in the city. These interests form an economic-commercial-political complex which comes to control the market place. Currently, citizens have become very interested in the quality of their own lives and are beginning to regard the community as a system to meet their needs. Purposes for their lives are being defined by them-

selves and their families. Purpose is a
particularly interesting question. What
is the purpose of Amherst? Is it to support a market place? Is it to support
this university? Community purposes are
usually not clearly defined and are often
different for different parts of the community.

One way to consider the matter is to
turn the market place/community relationship upside down and talk about the community as the purpose for the people who
live there--the community is a place for
life. The market place, instead of being
supported by the community, would support
the community. That has rather profound
implications, as can be imagined. For
example, it is now perfectly acceptable
to move company executives from town to
town; the city is there to support their
movement up through the organization and
their job is essentially to support that
enterprise. It would be a very different thing for the executives to be considered to have a basic commitment to the
community. They would probably not be
moved periodically.

An article that helped me understand
the community as a dynamic organization
was "The Local Community as an Ecology of
Games" by Norton Long (1958). He described
the community as a set of activities (games)
that play out simultaneously in time. They
have simultaneous interactions on the same
playing field. An individual may be playing in two or three different games at the
same time. He could be playing the family
game, the businessman's game, and the community leader's game. That is a useful

way to think about the community process,
the ways in which it gets organized, and
the rules by which each subpart is governed. Viewed as a system, the community is
quite differentiated in ways which have
been guided by the market place purpose,
and not differentiated in areas of human
need (e.g., for youth or the aged).

TECHNOLOGY OF COMMUNITY PSYCHOLOGY

Underlying the technology of community psychology is an ideology which is
an ecological one. It says one purpose
of life can be seen as getting into balance with the environment so that the best
possible life can be developed with the
minimum expenditure of nonreplaceable or
expensive energy. One can look around at
our society and see a system that is oriented differently. The industrial society
is a high-energy system with capital-in-
tensive means of production; it requires
increasingly smaller amounts of labor to
staff it. The energy consumed is largely
nonreplaceable. The rate of use has increased fantastically: more energy has
been used this century than all that was
used previously by man. This then indicates that the next hundred years hold
changes in the direction of lower energy
consumption and major changes in life
style (Meadows, Meadows, Randers, & Behrens, 1972).

There is a very interesting analog
to this energy perspective in higher education. We now think it to be appropriate to school people for a very long time
before they can be employed productively.
Most of the education is not directly re-

levant to the employment needs of the person. With this energy perspective in mind,
I reflected on a talk given by Ivan Illich
in Nashville about deschooling the society. I suddenly saw that Illich (1971) was
talking about institutions as an energy
matter. He observed that the life style
of the population of Mexico limits most
of the people to less than 20 miles from
their homes in the course of a month.
When they do go further, there is no particular hurry to get there. The loads
that they have to carry are relatively
small. He thought that their lives could
be conducted in Mexico (at the current
standards of living) with two engines, a
three-horsepower and a five-horsepower
engine. This line of thought was as a
direct analog to considering the function
of the school in society. Why are there
long periods of schooling (from 6-16 years
of age) and then no schooling program after that? There is a great lack of means
for personal development from the end of
one's schooling to his retirement. There
is a third-rate process called continuing
education, which seems to be oriented to
hobbies or to those people who can't find
a job. The resources for education seem
to be concentrated wrongly. Perhaps a
birth-to-death view of education which is
put into more purposeful chunks would make
most sense. Etzioni (1970) has a view of
the community as having a sizeable group
called the learning force which is related to the quality of life. Coleman
(1972) sees the school as having to be
restructured to provide meaningful participation of children and youth in the
urban community. Education and schooling may come to be very much more closely

related to the workplace than they currently are.

The energy perspective also helped me
to understand what George Miller (1969)
was saying in his APA Presidential address
about giving psychology away. The para-
professional movement took on new meaning.
It made me consider that the major investment in training doctoral journeymen is
too expensive in energy terms. We will
soon begin a major controversy in psychology over who are to be called psychologists and what is to be called psychology.

I discovered a book by Papanek (1971),
Design for the Real World, which illustrates all kinds of ways that human needs
can be met more cheaply. This, and the
Whole Earth Catalog (Portola Institute,
1971), have influenced me to try to design
lower-energy alternatives whenever possible. We had a chance to do this with a
project for the Tennessee Valley Authority. They were interested in the possibility of planning for Southern Tennessee
and Northern Alabama in a way which would
provide a new kind of "New Towns" development. They thought that New Towns should
be built around already extant villages
so that there would be a tradition from
which to build and so that the people
there would have a hand in shaping their
future. There was a little money, about
six or seven thousand dollars, to finance
a study of a number of communities to learn
about the residents' living preferences.
TVA wanted to know why the people lived
there, and how they would react to urban
services in what now is a rural area.

This project offered a challenge for
low-energy solutions. I wanted to see if
we could conduct a research project through
a community development process rather
than the usual strategy of taking in a team
of trained interviewers. We told the TVA
representative that the process would take
somewhat longer and that there might be
some negotiation with local community researchers about what got asked. If they
could tolerate those constraints in the
research, we would try to help. An agreement was developed. The role of the research group was defined as providing
technical assistance to the regional community development organization. We helped them hire two graduate students to do
field work and have proceeded, without
having university personnel take a primary role in the field. The development
association took the contract, hired the
staff, and supervised them. Our job was
to see that the research design, instruments, and procedures were appropriate.

RESEARCH IN COMMUNITY PSYCHOLOGY

Research and research training in
Community Psychology at Peabody College
has been developed and conducted mainly
in the Center for Community Studies (Newbrough, Rhodes, & Seeman, 1970). Research
projects have typically been generated to
serve programmatic interests in the community and at the same time to be approached
theoretically to serve training needs.
The Center's board, in 1967, realized that
there was a basic lack of sustained research into the effects of community change
on the various types of residents. There
was no way to fit together the different

community research projects nor to assess
the effects of community action projects.

The Center began developing a community change research program. A conference was held (with NIMH funding) in 1970
to consider the development of local social indicators in health, education, and
housing (Center for Community Studies,
1970). In 1971-73, the Center participated with the Urban Observatory of Metropolitan Nashville-University Centers
in the collection of social indicators
for a local social report. In 1971, the
Center also participated with the Center
for Epidemiologic Studies, NIMH, in planning for a collaborative study of depressed mood in local community settings.
This led to the receipt of a two-year
developmental grant from the Center for
Epidemiologic Studies to produce a plan
and the instrumentation for it. This
project, Community Mental Health Epidemiology (MH20681) was not designed to be
a standard population study of the incidence and prevalence of cases, but was
oriented to repeated measurements on a
population for a condition which all persons have--mood. Thus, we turned this
epidemiological project toward normal life
processes and the ways that they are influenced by the functioning of the organized community.[1]

---

[1]Detailed information on the CMHE
project is available from the author, Center for Community Studies, Peabody College,
Box 319, Nashville, Tennessee 37203

The early interests from NIMH were
in the monitoring of mood weekly to see
whether events would be related to it, and
whether one could detect sufficient rises
and falls to see "epidemics" of depressed
mood. My own interests were in the functioning of the organized community to help
and impede coping of individuals with life
stress events, and whether social role
functioning related in any direct way with
the presence of psychiatric symptoms. I
personally believed the case-oriented concern with symptoms and syndromes to be a
fruitless way of searching for the mentally disordered. Rather, if one wished
to find the people who required mental
health services, we should look for people who were not fulfilling social roles
or who were under some stress. We tried
to integrate these two views.

As one gets into a monitoring study
the need for theory becomes clear, particularly when one proposes to collect data
at differing levels of analysis and at
differing places in the community. We
developed a three-level theory to help us
select variables. At the most global
level, we wished to consider the relationship of community processes and events
to mood in the population. At a lower level, we wished to consider the impacts of
community processes and events on relationships of persons to their life settings. At the third level, we were interested in the impacts of community processes and events upon individuals' levels
of depressed mood.

The community was defined as the
political-geographic unit of Nashville.

The government is organized to serve a
particular area. It gets its resources,
at least in part, from that area; the
channels for the people to participate in
the system are established. The community is organized in various forms to meet
individual needs. The services and resources are distributed in particular
ways which yield differential need-meeting. Of particular interest is whether
depressed mood (and other mood reactions)
will be indicative of failures in meeting
needs in or by the community.

The theory is arranged around the
central construct of mood which is affected by two things: events and need-
meeting. That is, variables with vary-
ing reactivity to community changes interact to yield mood. In order to study
short-term variation, the population was
sampled weekly. The NIMH was in the field
in Kansas City and in Washington County
(Hagerstown), Maryland, for the year of
1972, and has weekly data for that period. This schedule turned out to be too
difficult. The weekly samples of 25-30
were too small with too much variation
between them. The pressure on the sur-
veying staff was relentless and often more
than they could deal with. We decided to
use monthly sampling. This was bolstered
by our theoretical view that depressed
mood should last 4-8 weeks after the pre-
cipitating event (as hypothesized by Gerald Caplan's crisis theory--personal communication, 1960). A new sample will be
opened every month with a follow-up on
that sample for three successive months.
Each sample of 200 will stand as a representative sample of the community and will

yield a short-term panel. In any given
month we will have estimates of the community mood from four different probabi-
lity samples (one original and three at
different stages of follow-up). These 800
subjects will greatly augment the confidence that we will be willing to attach to
findings.

Community data will be collected on
a monthly basis. The aspects of the community samples are variables to reflect
(1) reactivity to events (the most short
term), (2) resources and their allocation
(probably changing yearly), and (3) integration of the total community (changing
slowly over several years). Short-term
variables are those like demands on service. If there is an event that sends
people for service, that should show up
in the data. Other examples of short-term
need-meeting are admissions to emergency
wards, presentations to mental health
clinics, and calls to the crisis center.
One variable we particularly want is complaints. Our theory holds that complaining behavior is extraordinarily important
to the relationship of the person in his
community. It is thought to occur prior
to turning negative feelings inward and
becoming alienated or depressed. There
is no good way of getting an overall measure of complaining behavior in the community. We will have to develop these measures. A few strictly environmental measures such as weather are believed to affect mood (Helsing, 1973). One interesting finding reported to us was that when
a weather front passes through, children
in school are more irritable and behaviorally active (Willard Smith, personal com-

munication). When the wind blows in
Northern California, there seems to be a
relationship with presentations to the
mental health clinics (Captane Thompson,
personal communication). These suggest
intriguing kinds of ebbs and flows of behavior that go along with weather. The
community data are collected monthly,
managed on the computer, and displayed
graphically by means of the Community Information System.

What will the data look like? While
leafing through Forrester's book, Industrial Dynamics (1961), I found some figures that looked like EEG write-outs.
There were several variables all rising
and falling in relation to a time line,
and to each other. The analogy is direct
with our plans for the display of time
series data. With such a display of mood
and community variables, one will want
to know what the usual variations (base
rates) are so that an unusual deflection
can be identified. When the calibrations
are completed, then one has the problem
of explaining the variation. The first
thing is to see whether two or more variables seem to be related. If they are
reliably related, one can start the development of hypotheses about how they are
related. There is a further interesting
problem of leads and lags of relationships.
A helpful approach to this problem is Jay
Forrester's work on systems modelling.
The book on industrial dynamics shows how
one can look at the rises and falls in a
factory's inventory system. As one studies it, the factory application shows
how some rises lead to others; and they make
intuitive sense. The community is not a

factory; we do not know the interrelation-
ships of variables. Thus, if we find that
events and mood are related temporally to
each other, we can then set about explor-
ing the causal linkages.

One of the major problems in the study is to define an event. We have considered mood in an Adaptation Level theory
perspective where one has an organism
adapting itself to an environment, cen-
tering around some stimuli. When center-
ing or stabilization has occurred, the organism then attends to stimuli which break
through some sort of adaptation level and
which often call for some behavioral response. Changes or shifts in life circumstances usually stimulate major affective
reactions. Stress, in this context, is
basically a disjunction between the person and environment. What is stressful
is the amount of disjunction and the amount
of work the organism has to go through to
re-center. We began to view depressed
mood as a mood which follows anxiety as a
residual matter and cumulates into a feeling with a longer duration. It is somewhat less sensitive to the immediate situation and is a moderate-term affective
state. Depressed mood is regarded as happening to everybody. I see it as the re-
fractory phase of the adaptation, following the initial response of anxiety.

The measurement of depressed mood as
a phenomenon is a particularly problema-
tic matter. It requires self-reporting
which is done (a) as answers to structured
interview questions; (2) as responses to
standard psychological tests; or (3) as
the reporting on the person by a signifi-

cant other. The state of the art is primitive. The CMHE project began some work on the development of a scale which has major needs for work on reliability and validity. We did some work in Norwich, Connecticut (with the Psychiatric Epidemiology Research Unit, Poughkeepsie, New York) and in Nashville, Tennessee, this past year to explore the problem. The NIMH has data on some additional scales in their two field sites.[2] The major problem, however, has to do with the criterion of **when** is mood depressed and **how much**?

Relationships with local community have been of particular interest to us (1) from the perspective of maintaining our ability to do monitoring research over a five-year period, and (2) from our ideology that research data should be translated into information and utilized as widely as possible. At the beginning of the project we established a standing committee, the Committee of Collaborators, which has about 20 members from the mental health centers, state departments of mental health and health, university departments, local health department, and the like. This group will begin to operate as an active users group when the project is operational.

One of our basic concerns has been the protection of privacy of our respondents. As a basic office procedure, we

---

[2]For information about this write to Robert Markush, M.D., Chief, Center for Epidemiologic Studies, NIMH, 5600 Fishers Lane, Rockville, Maryland 20852

have designed a name coding procedure to
remove names from all research materials.
We have invited a member of the local American Civil Liberties Union Chapter to be
on the committee to monitor the project
and its procedures. The larger implications of the data as a management information resource at the community level have
not been thought through in detail; but we
do see potential social control problems
where the mayor or police chief may wish
to use the information for superficial
reasons.

EPILOGUE

This kind of research is, in my view,
an example of what I think community psychology to be all about. Here is a phenomenon approached at several levels of
discourse. My own inclination has been
to look at these levels, as starting from
the person and going up into the community
system. This keeps me focused on the issue of the quality of life in the houses
and in the work places in the community.
In the end, I would hope that systems will
be much more concerned about the persons
who run them and who get served by them.
One of the major anxieties that I have is
that this study may be ahead of its time
in the sense that the legal safeguards
are not in place. It has even led me to
wonder whether the research plan should
be merely written up and allowed to sit
for several years until the social situation is much more stable and less concerned with deviant behavior.

An interesting aspect of this study
is that it takes psychology up to a higher

level of abstraction than the discipline
has been comfortable with. We have involved persons and knowledge from economics, political science, sociology, public health, demography, and the like;
something not usually done in the halls
of psychology. We can, as psychologists
in concert with other colleagues, address
some of the critical issues of the future,
such as the design of habitats and environments, and the effects of lifestyles
and living arrangements on behavior. We
can also begin to think about low-energy
alternatives for solution of problems and
we can begin to explore whether it is possible to design for a voluntary society
(Schindler-Rainman & Lippitt, 1971). Perhaps the major problem in America today is
one of culture lag. It is very easy, in
the short run, for us to think that change
agentry is the matter that psychology practice and training should be directed to.
This would help to ease the culture lag
changes. I think that we must look beyond
the notion of change agent since it has
no clear meaning in relationship to the
macrosystem. We have to address the question of change _for_ _what_ _purpose_? I am
very dubious of community psychology es-
pousing change agentry as a technology
without a purposeful philosophy associ-
ated with it.

I see community psychology as a sci-
entifically-based movement, but one which
will also incorporate a strong applied
aspect to it. Rather than the two-sided
dichotomy of the Boulder model of the
scientist-professional, I see the community psychologist being trained to do
systematic inquiry in his regular work

places with an emphasis on dissemination and utilization of the knowledge generated. There will be science and profession aspects but these will be integrated; he will not have to pay separate homage to each. I would suspect that two things will happen that will profoundly affect psychology and science:

1) community psychology will force psychology to be more holistic, environmentally oriented, and concerned with futures, and
2) community psychology will bring together interdisciplinary groups and approach the solving of community and social problems by a mix of perspectives and methods.

REFERENCES

Allport, F. Theories of perception and the concept of structure. New York: Wiley, 1955.

Bauer, R. N + 1 ways not to run a railroad. American Psychologist, 1960, 15, 650-655.

Bennett, C. C. et al. Community psychology: A report of the Boston conference on the education of psychologists for community mental health. Boston: Boston University, 1966.

Bentley, A. F. The human skin: Philosophy's last line of defense. Philosophy of Science, 1941, 8, 1-19.

Bentley, A. F. Kennetic inquiry. Science,

1950, 112, 775-783.

Cantril, H. The morning notes of Adelbert Ames, Jr. New Brunswick, N.J.: Rutgers University Press, 1960.

Center for Community Studies. Social change and quality of life: A report on a conference held in Nashville, Tennessee, May 7-9, 1970. Nashville: Center for Community Studies, 1970. (A final grant report submitted to the Center for Studies of Metropolitan Problems, NIMH.)

Coleman, J. Our children have outgrown the schools. Psychology Today, 1972, 5(9), 72-75.

Denzin, N. The research act. Chicago: Aldine, 1970.

Dewey, J., & Bentley, A. F. Knowing and the known. Boston: Beacon Press, 1949.

Etzioni, A. Indicators of the capacity for societal guidance. The Annals of the American Academy of Political and Social Science, 1970, 388, 25-34.

Forrester, J. W. Industrial dynamics. Cambridge, Mass.: MIT Press, 1961.

Golann, S. E. Coordinate index reference guide to community mental health. New York: Behavioral Publications, 1969.

Gordon, T. Parent effectiveness training. New York: Wyden, 1970.

Harris, T. A. I'm ok; you're ok. New

York: Avon Books, 1973.

Helsing, K. J. Weather and mood. Working Paper #41, January 1973. Community
Mental Health Epidemiology: Collaborative Study, MH20681-02, National Insti-
tue of Mental Health.

Hofstader, R. Social Darwinism in American thought. Boston: Beacon Press,
1970.

Illich, I. Deschooling society. New
York: Harper & Row, 1971.

Levin, H. Psychologist for the powerless.
In F. F. Korten, S. W. Cook, & J. I.
Lacey (Eds.) Psychology and the problems
of society. Washington, D.C.: American Psychological Association, 1970.

Long, N. The local community as an ecology of games. The American Sociological Review, 1958, 64, 251-261.

Massachusetts General Hospital and Harvard Medical School. Community mental
health and social psychiatry: A reference guide. Cambridge, Mass.: Harvard
University Press, 1963.

Meadows, D. H., Meadows, D. L., Randers,
J., & Behrens, W. W., III. The limits
to growth: A report for the Club of
Rome's project on the predicament of
mankind. New York: Universe Books,
1972.

Michael, D. Cybernation: The silent
conquest. Santa Barbara, Calif.: Center for the Study of Democratic Institu-

tions, 1962.

Miller, G. A. Psychology as a means for promoting human welfare. American Psychologist, 1969, 24, 1063-1075.

Morris, C. Signs, language and behavior. New York: Prentice-Hall, 1946.

Newbrough, J. R. The resource person in the community: A method for evaluating the reporter's reports. Mental Health Study Center, National Institute of Mental Health, 1965. Mimeo.

Newbrough, J. R. Comment on S. Lehmann's article: Community, psychology, and community psychology. American Psychologist, 1972, 27, 770-772.

Newbrough, J. R., Rhodes, W. C., & Seeman, J. The development of community psychology at George Peabody College. In I. Iscoe & C. Spielberger (Eds.) Community psychology: Perspectives in training and research. New York: Appleton-Century-Crofts, 1970.

Papanek, V. Design for the real world: Human ecology and social change. New York: Pantheon, 1971.

Portola Institute. The last whole earth catalog. New York: Random House, 1971.

Rawls, J. A theory of justice. Cambridge, Mass.: Harvard University, 1971.

Reiff, R. Psychology and public policy. Professional Psychology, 1970, 1(4), 315-324.

Revel, J. F.   Without Marx or Jesus.
Saturday Review, 1971, 54, 14-31.

Rousseau, J. J.   The social contract, or
principles of political right.   New
York: E. B. Dutton & Company, 1913.

Sanford, N.   Whatever happened to action
research?   Journal of Social Issues,
1970, 26(4), 3-23.

Schindler-Rainman, E., & Lippitt, R.   The
volunteer community: Creative use of
human resources.   Washington, D.C.:
NTL Institute of Applied Behavioral Sciences, 1971.

U. S. National Institute of Mental Health.
Evaluation in mental health: A review
of the problem of evaluating mental
health activities.   Washington, D. C.:
U.S.G.P.O., 1955.

von Bertalanffy, L.   General systems theory.   New York: Braziller, 1968.

Webb, E. J., Campbell, D. T., Schwartz,
R. D. & Sechrist, L.   Unobtrusive measures: Nonreactive research in the social sciences.   Chicago: Rand McNally,
1966.

Weber, M.   Nature of the city.   In R. Warren (Ed.) Perspectives on the American
community: A book of readings.   Chicago:
Rand McNally, 1966.

Wheeler, H.   Democracy in a revolutionary
era.   Santa Barbara, Calif.:   The Center
for the Study of Democratic Institutions,
1968.

2. COLLABORATIVE INTERVENTIONS IN COMMUNITY MENTAL HEALTH: A PERSONAL PERSPECTIVE

Jack M. Chinsky

The purpose of this paper is to describe my professional involvement in the field of community psychology. It includes a brief historical account of my developing interest in the area, a description of my current activities, and my views on the future of the discipline. The paper is meant to reflect a personal perspective and is not intended to define or review the broad and complex scope of the field.

ANTECEDENTS

My work in community psychology "officially" began in 1967 and, in retrospect, extended from three sources. The first could best be described as the general climate of social activism in the sixties. The campus was a center of political interest and activity and I and many of my fellow students were engaged in some form of political action. Social problems, e.g.,

poverty, prejudice, inequalities in education, etc., were highly visible. Riot-
ing had occurred in many cities including
Rochester, New York, where I was attending graduate school, and in Newark, near
my home. The exposure of these problems
produced a sense of despair, on the one
hand, but also a strong sense of hope.
The "Great Society" was still a possibility and the youth movement was an important part of the process. There was a growing notion that maybe at this moment of
social awareness and untapped potential
we really could "change the system."

The second influence was my growing
dissatisfaction with the state of psychology as it was currently practiced. My
initial training in graduate school primarily emphasized the traditional approaches to diagnosis and therapy. Alternative and more active approaches were
looked at unfavorably. Even behavior
modification was considered a fairly ra-
dical approach and when I or a fellow
student advocated a behavioral perspective, we were derisively labeled "behavioral engineers" or "plumbers."

The problem was highlighted by the
fact that as interns we neither had the
background in psychotherapy to know what
we were doing nor were we given the most
desirable clients, the ones who would be
the best motivated and most appropriate
for traditional psychotherapeutic techniques. Given these conditions, we were
quite limited in what we were allowed to
do.

Two cases that I had at the time illustrate the point. I was working with a
Black thirteen-year-old at Rochester State
Hospital. The goal of treatment was to
provide this youngster with the skills
necessary for adequate interpersonal relations. My major contact with him occurred once or twice a week for an hour in
the framework of verbally-oriented therapy. At the same time, I visited his home
in the ghetto and knew that even if I
achieved everything I wanted to and helped this child to develop a minimal level
of social skills, he would be returning
to an environment that would challenge
even the most adaptively functioning
adult. The whole approach seemed dras-
tically shortsighted and futile.

The other case was an adult female
client who had been diagnosed as a manic-
depressive and had improved to the point
of wanting to get a job in the community.
Being sort of untraditional even at that
time, I tried to help her get the job and
discovered that this was impossible because she was listed by potential employ-
ers as a former state hospital patient.
It seemed as if the patient and I were up
against a brick wall. How do you help
people achieve adequate self-esteem when
they must interact in a society working
against that purpose?

Again, I felt very limited. It seemed that I was being taught to use old
techniques for new clients with new goals.
Our clients were extending beyond the
population of young, attractive, verbal,
intelligent, successful, middle class,
white neurotics, but our treatment ap-

proaches were not (Schofield, 1964). The
field was, to use Golann's (1970) framework, profession-helper oriented. Intervention was geared to the skills already
in the practitioner's repertoire rather
than the needs of the client.

Community psychology, which had just
become officially organized, had a great
appeal to me. It was active rather than
passive, system oriented rather than individual oriented, behavioral rather than
verbal, and preventative rather than rehabilitative. Perhaps most important,
it was optimistic and hopeful rather than
irrelevant to the goals and challenges
that I was encountering.

The third major influence was my association with Julian Rappaport and Emory
L. Cowen at the University of Rochester.
Cowen was the director of the clinical
program and actively engaged in community
psychology. Rappaport was a close friend
and fellow classmate who had the idea of
following up the Poser (1966) study using
college students as nonprofessional therapeutic agents in a mental hospital. It
was the support and encouragement of these
men that channeled my developing interest
in the field into a concrete project.

THE ROCHESTER STATE HOSPITAL PROJECT

Rappaport's idea was so intriguing
that I dropped my plans to conduct a dissertation in clinical-developmental psychology and moved into this very new area
of community mental health. The project
at Rochester State Hospital is described

in detail in <u>Innovations in Helping Chronic Patients: College Students in a Mental Institution</u> (Rappaport, Chinsky, & Cowen, 1971) and will be discussed only briefly here.

Undergraduates from the University of Rochester worked with groups of eight chronic patients, meeting with them twice weekly for about five months. The general goal of the program was to energize and increase the social skills of the patients through interaction with enthusiastic, flexible, and sensitive college students. The project was large and difficult with 256 patients in our initial treatment group. Along with our 64 controls, just about every back ward patient between the ages of 21 and 59 who had been in the hospital more than a year and could write his or her name was involved in the program.

Many of my gains from the intervention were personal. These included the friendships I found with the students, patients, and staff, as well as the sense of accomplishment at seeing the project become reality. Equally important was the satisfaction of seeing improvement and growth in both the students and patients.

At the same time, I was given a first-rate education on the functioning of the institution itself; we later termed the institution "The Sleeping Dragon" (Rappaport, Chinsky, & Cowen, 1971). Rappaport and I were interns at the hospital; our primary, traditional responsibilities were focused on the newer, acute units,

especially the children's wards. There
was a remarkable contrast between the
conditions in these units and the back
wards where our project was conducted.
Small gains, such as securing approximately $90 per week for overtime staff
to help bring the 256 patients to the
companion groups twice a week, were seen
as major accomplishments.

Some of our work made it necessary
to be on the back wards after the usual
five o'clock exodus of the professional
staff. It was not atypical during these
later hours to find one attendant respon-
sible for more than seventy patients. One
way the attendants dealt with this inadequate staff/patient ratio was to put the
patients to sleep at seven o'clock or
seven thirty. The lights were turned off
and patients were told that all recrea-
tional activities were over. Getting the
patients to sleep at that hour was greatly aided by the overly large doses of
thorazine and other mind-dulling drugs.
Other experiences such as witnessing the
"cattle-like" atmosphere in the halls or
having to pick a patient up from his own
pool of urine to be brought to a group
convinced me that institutional change
was a top priority for psychologists.

The Rochester State Hospital project
was researched in the form of a joint dissertation. Rappaport and I had separate
research proposals, committee meetings,
written theses, and orals, but the intervention was combined in practice. I focused on the research issues involving
the college students (Chinsky, 1968) and
Rappaport (1968) focused on the patients.

The program was designed, implemented,
and evaluated between January, 1967, and
the summer of 1968, a few weeks before my
beginning an appointment at the University
of Connecticut in Storrs.

NONPROFESSIONAL THERAPEUTIC ATTRIBUTES

The teaching-research position at
Connecticut began for me a process of
professional identification which is still
continuing and changing. As noted above,
my own training, except for the last one-
and-a-half years, was fairly traditional,
yet at Connecticut, I was viewed in the
role of <u>the</u> community psychologist. I had
to determine what my relationship was to
clinical psychology as well as where I
fit specifically in the broader and more
nebulous area of community psychology.

My research since the dissertation
has followed two lines of general interest. The first encompasses a direct extension of my work on so-called nonprofessional therapeutic attributes, basic
human skills that relate to effectiveness
in dealing with other people. While conceptualizing the dissertation, I recognized that the global term "nonprofessional" was too broad to describe a group of
treatment agents with so many varied
skills and abilities. Kiesler (1966) has
stressed the same criticism of the undif-
ferentiated term "psychotherapists" in
more traditional psychotherapy research.

Not all nonprofessionals are equally
effective; some may be harmful for certain clients. One of the primary con-

cerns in nonprofessional programs is to
determine selection procedures that as-
sure choosing the most suitable therapeutic workers. This question is of special importance in these programs for
two reasons. First, nonprofessionals are
usually drawn from a more diverse population than professionals and seldom en-
counter the rigorous admission procedures
or lengthy program requirements that fos-
ter a high degree of self-selection. Second, nonprofessional programs tend to re-
ly less on training than on selection.
Training, when it occurs, is usually found
within the ongoing intervention. Programs
tend to be shorter and more goal-specific
than the rigorous four- to six-year learning and weeding process that precedes professional credentials.

One of the major aspects of my work
in this area is the continued application
and development of the Group Assessment
of Interpersonal Traits (GAIT), a simu-
lated group interaction technique first
developed by Goodman (1972). The GAIT
was the only measure of nonprofessional
attributes--and the only behavioral de-
vice--that had even a modest relationship
to independent indices of patient improvement in my dissertation. None of the
other fifty scales used in that study, including Accurate Empathy (Truax & Carkhuff, 1967) and the AB dimension (Whitehorn & Betz, 1954), correlated significantly with patient change.

A GAIT group is composed of six to
eight participants who are asked to engage
in a series of dyadic relationships. One
group member is encouraged to disclose a

personal problem and another takes the
role of trying to understand that problem. It is a fairly stressful procedure involving a great deal of disclosure
and sharing. Participants are rated behaviorally on the dimensions of "open-
ness," "understanding," and "warmth."

I have continued to use the GAIT in
subsequent nonprofessional programs.
The measure has also proved useful in research on the composition and evaluation
of sensitivity groups (D'Augelli & Chinsky, in press). People rated high on the
GAIT dimensions, for example, have been
found to engage in more personal feedback
and disclosure in later t-group interactions (D'Augelli, Chinsky, & Getter, in
press). It appears that the same willingness and ability to assume "therapeutic"
social roles are important in both sensitivity training and a number of companionship programs. These skills are fairly
complex, and recent studies have shown
that simple instruction alone is not sufficient to elicit them (D'Augelli & Chinsky, in press). I have also been examining the therapeutic qualities of understanding (Bambrough, 1973) and self-dis-
closure (Ansama, 1974) in other studies
besides those using the GAIT.

COMMUNITY MENTAL HEALTH PROGRAMS

The second, related area of my interest has been in the implementation and
evaluation of new community projects. It
is essentially this work which most clearly defines my current role in the field.
I would like to present this aspect of my

work in the following sequence. First, I
am going to describe the model of intervention that I use in these projects--the
"collaborative intervention design." Second, I will share some personal perspectives about community mental health programs in general, especially those elements of these projects that are not usually discussed in the literature but are
crucial to their success. Third, I will
focus on a concrete description of those
interventions with which I have worked.
Finally, I will illustrate how my participation in these projects defines my present place in the community movement.

The Collaborative Intervention Design

The University of Connecticut offers
an eclectic clinical training program
which is supportive but not solely oriented toward community psychology. I do
not have the luxury of a full-scale community program with a sequence of courses
or four or five professors focusing on
the area. Students obtain their Ph.D.'s
in clinical psychology and the majority
do not spend all of their efforts in community.

The collaborative intervention design or "mental health quarterback model"
(Cowen, 1967; Cowen, Chinsky, & Rappaport,
1970), which was so useful for me at the
University of Rochester seemed ideal for
this graduate program as well. The model,
in its most basic form, consists of a professional who consults with graduate students. The graduate students, in turn,
supervise a team of undergraduates who
serve as direct service agents. The de-

sign was given its original name because
it allows the professional, by coordinating this network, to extend the scope of
his outreach almost geometrically. The
effectiveness of the model (see Table 1)
requires special roles for each member of
the collaborative intervention team as
well as a specific relationship between
this team and the community group or institution with which they are working.

My primary role as the professional
is that of a consultant coordinating all
aspects of the program. I frequently work
with another faculty member at this level
to share the time load and add the skills
he has to offer. A great deal of my work
involves supervision of the graduate students.

The graduate student, supervising
undergraduates and working with a community agency, learns not only how to implement and evaluate an intervention, but
also a variety of administrative and consultative techniques. The latter skills
are extremely important for the contemporary professional psychologist (Rotter,
1973).

I encourage the graduate students to
work together either simultaneously or in
sequence. A single master's thesis or
Ph.D. dissertation is seldom broad enough
to encompass a meaningful community intervention. Several projects conducted simultaneously allow the broadened scope
and depth that these programs require.
Sequential projects offer the continuity
also necessary for these programs. I try
to support the interest of new students in

TABLE 1
SCHEMATIZATION OF THE COLLABORATIVE INTERVENTION DESIGN

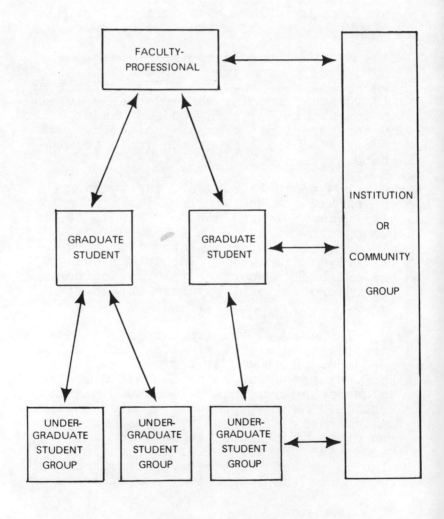

TABLE 2

OUTLINE OF THE MULTILEVEL INTERVENTION PROGRAM IN AN ELEMENTARY SCHOOL

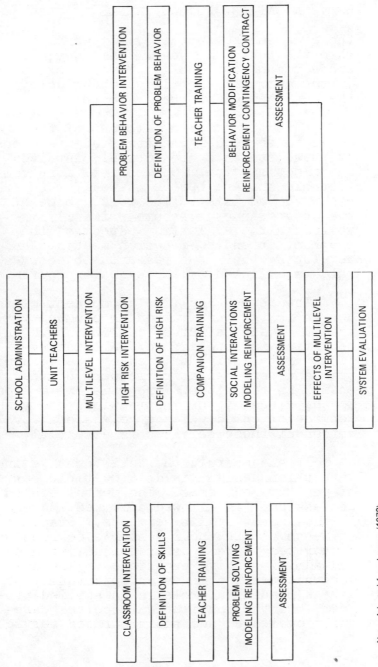

Note: Adapted from Larcen (1973).

the programs so that they may work with
them the following year. This way, a
project can continue for five or six years
in the community setting without delaying
the advancement of the graduate student.

A third and vital element of the
model is the undergraduate students. Most
of these students are actively involved
in direct service. Others feel more comfortable and are better suited for supervisory or administrative work. Some of
the undergraduates become primarily involved in the evaluation aspect of the
program, attending research meetings and
developing their own research objectives
which are linked to the overall program.

The fourth and final component of the
design is the institution or community
group. Again, a mutual collaborative interaction is established. All interventions are jointly designed by the academic
team and representative members of the
social institutions. Programs are geared
to the needs of the institutions and are
service oriented; of course, careful evaluation of these services is essential.

If successful, the collaborative intervention design yields a multiple series
of positive outcomes. The mental health
professional is allowed a marked increase
in the impact of his services. Graduate
students obtain their master's degrees or
doctorates as well as practical research
and administrative experience. The undergraduates are given an opportunity to
have a meaningful role in an applied program, and the institution receives carefully evaluated and administrated services.

The design also has unique advantages for
both the training of psychologists (Rotter, 1973) and the alleviation of mental
health manpower shortages in the field
(Albee, 1967).

The model conforms to Rotter's (1973)
suggestion on the training of clinical
psychologists because the professional
and the graduate students under his supervision are diagnosing the needs of the
social system and carefully evaluating
the intervention. The nonprofessionals
whom they train are performing the bulk
of the direct service role. The model is
also a practicable solution to the professional manpower shortage as it markedly increases the range of a single professional's contact.

Special Features of Community Programs

Perhaps one of the most important
but least considered aspects of this form
of community intervention is the role of
personal enthusiasm and motivation. Of
course, all good research demands a great
deal of work and endurance, but these qualities are especially important in community studies. Research on practical social problems generally takes more time
and effort, and relies more on personal
contact than most laboratory studies. At
the same time, variables are less easily
controlled, results are less clear, and
the security of completion of the project
is generally less certain. In addition
to these problems, community researchers
are frequently under attack by their academic colleagues for not being scientific
enough and by the community members for

not being service oriented enough.

Thus, personal zeal is not simply a beneficial accompaniment to these projects but a vital element. Two essential factors serve to enhance and maintain this enthusiasm. The first is the novelty and innovativeness of community projects. Research meetings are sometimes the most exciting focus for this crusading spirit. Many hours are frequently spent in groups that look like the strategy room meetings of a "grade B" war movie. Research plans and terms fit well into a form of battle analogue. For example, there are several "fronts" with which we have to work, such as the university and the community groups. Undergraduates are at the "front lines," etc. Blackboards and pads of paper are filled with calendars and flow charts outlining the next steps to be taken in the project.

This "intensity of initiation" can be maintained over years if the project continues to evolve and grow. Change, itself, must be built into the program. I have seldom seen a student or other community worker content to be a nonprofessional for more than two years. Changing roles is made relatively easy using the collaborative intervention design because, except for myself and the institution, all of the other staff people are moving on.

The greatest danger in these types of programs is institutionalization. If the project is allowed to become stagnant and bureaucratic, goals shift from those of the original intervention to the maintenance of the program per se. The members

of the staff become more interested in
knowing how jobs are going to be kept and
salaries raised than how much they are ac-
complishing. The different orientations
can best be summarized by the contrasting
concerns "How are you going to put yourself
out of business?" to that of "How are you
going to perpetuate the business?"

This institutionalization process may
account for some of the problems that are
seen in programs of a national scope, such
as Headstart. Headstart began with a good
idea and a group of personally motivated
people dedicated to the goals of the program. The notion of mass producing the
project, generalizing from one setting to
another, giving money, and saying "Do
Headstart" did not, however, convey the
kind of personal enthusiasm that was inherent in the success of the original project. This expansion also reduced the appreciation for the complexities of this
form of program such as the subsequent
continuation by local school systems and
a variety of socioeconomic problems that
would also have to be addressed.

The second major factor necessary to
maintain the zeal of these projects is
the selection of personnel. Undergraduates are relatively easy to find; there
are many more of them and they often tend
to have more enthusiasm than graduate
students. Most graduate programs do not
select students on the basis of skills
necessary to conduct community interventions (Kelly, 1970). One factor that may
affect this selection problem is the importance placed on academic criteria sometimes at the expense of social skills.

If a department focuses exclusively on
grades they may get a group of students
less willing or unable to work in the community. As mentioned above, such programs
require more effort and risk taking as
well as an increased reliance on interpersonal skills than more traditional research. Selecting graduate students and
undergraduates who are personally commit-
ted to the program and share its enthusiasm and excitement ensures that even the
most difficult and ambitious intervention
has the spirit necessary for success.

There are three other features of
community programs that I would like to
stress. One of them is the uniqueness of
most of these projects. Even though they
might look quite similar on paper, programs can be very different depending on
the setting, the time, and the personalities involved. These idiographic elements make it extremely important for the
investigator to know the system in which
he is working. Understanding and appre-
ciating the subtleties of a particular
setting sometimes requires years of prior
contact before the intervention can be
attempted.

Time alone is often not enough. There
are projects that could be conducted in a
semirural setting in Connecticut that
would be impossible in New York City and
vice versa. We have been able to develop
a project in one school involving the entire student body and staff over the course
of a full year, but can't get in the front
door of a school less than a hundred yards
away.

These idiosyncratic features of community programs work counter to quick
generalizations about successful approaches
and simple solutions to social problems.
Along these lines, an adequate description
of the social system in which the program
was conducted is extremely important in
any research reports of these projects.
Such descriptions allow for a richer and
clearer understanding of these programs
and enhance the possibility that they may
be properly replicated.

A second point very much related to
the uniqueness of the program is the importance of personal relationships. Successful programs can seldom be implemented without a great deal of personal interaction with the community group or institution with which you are working. Mutual
trust and open communication are vital
factors in any intervention and there is
no shortcut to these ends. Some programs
take years of interaction preceding the
intervention to ensure that the investigator not only knows the system well, but
has established these personal bonds.

The final element necessary for a
successful community mental health intervention is to promote the building of resources within the social system that you
are working with. This allows the investigator the freedom of altering the intervention or even terminating it while the
program operations are continued by the
system itself. This mode of intervention
also reduces the agency's dependence on
an outsider and thus supports self-reli-
ance. Sometimes external support programs
serve to delay the need for making impor-

tant internal changes. For example, providing health services from an outside
project might delay the development of
these facilities within the local area.

A Preschool Education Program

        The first project that I initiated
at the University of Connecticut was a
preschool intervention for Puerto Rican
children and their families. The program
was conducted over a three-year period.
I worked with a graduate student the first
year, another graduate student the second,
and an undergraduate supervisory group the
third. Our goal was to help the children
develop increased competence in intellectual and social skills as well as to work
with their families in obtaining adequate
legal, social, and medical services.

        My initial contact for the program
was the director of the local Headstart
agency who had some Puerto Rican children
in her program and knew of many others in
need of such services who could not be
accommodated. Further, literature in the
field suggested that Headstart did not intervene early enough nor was it sufficiently extensive to be maximally beneficial to the children. Other programs
working with younger children had shown
more positive results.

        I was eager to begin an intervention
in Connecticut and this seemed an ideal
starting point. I was especially enthusiastic because my last project had used
nonprofessionals in a tertiary prevention
framework with chronic patients. I was
sure that nonprofessionals would be equal-

ly effective at the other end of the spec-
trum in a program with a primary prevention focus. Local community leaders were
contacted; they acknowledged that such a
program was needed and agreed to help in
its design and implementation.

Our service agents were undergraduate
women who were fluent in Spanish, liked
children, and had the necessary interpersonal skills. We selected our undergraduates not only from the University of
Connecticut but also from a local college
in line with my desire to reduce institutional boundaries wherever possible.
About a third of our "tutor-companions,"
as they were called, were Puerto Ricans;
half were from a Spanish-speaking country. The others became fluent in Spanish
after taking a number of Spanish language
courses. The final selection of these women was done with the help of a few community people. One of the criteria for
selection was that the tutor-companion
would have to be able to relate comfort-
ably with these people and convince them
of her personal commitment to the project.
The community representatives had a veto
and if they felt that a woman would not
be able to hack it, they told us.

The tutor-companions worked five days
a week for an hour in the children's homes.
The interaction with the children, who
ranged in age from 21 to 47 months, included a variety of tasks. The emphasis
was on having the children and tutor-companions enjoy their relationship as much
as possible. The undergraduates brought
in educational toys and began teaching
language and cognitive development. In

addition, they took the children on trips,
went shopping with them, and, in general,
tried to increase their experiential
world.

Most of the conversation was in Spanish in accord with the parents' wishes.
We did not attempt to teach the children
English unless it was requested. It was
not our aim to impose the Anglo culture
or language on the people.

At the same time that the college women tutored the children, they acted as
companions with the families. Adult family members were strongly encouraged to
participate in the tutoring relationship
and siblings were welcomed. Many of the
students became quite close to the families and shared dinners, trips, and holi-
days. They also served as translators
and advocates helping to secure needed
services.

I considered the program effective
both from a traditional research perspective as well as a humanistic one. Several
children received necessary medical care
including proper diets for nutritional
deficiency. Other problems, such as housing, jobs, and welfare, were also dealt
with.

One incident with housing illustrates
how complicated and involving research in
this area can be. We had previously divided up the city into experimental and
control areas to prevent confounding of
our treatment effects. When the house at
one of our experimental families burned,
we actually had to help them relocate in

an experiemtnal neighborhood.

In accord with our intellectual and
social objectives, some of the children
were given not just a headstart, but a
"head and shoulders" start into the schools.
A few of these gains were reflected at the
appropriate significance levels on measures
of vocabulary and intelligence.

Despite these positive outcomes, I
was not completely satisfied with the intervention over the three years. One of
the major difficulties of the program was
the enormous amount of time meeded for
routine administrative tasks. Maintenance issues, such as coordinating sche-
dules and arranging carpools, sometimes
had to take precedence over both the service and research aspects of the project.

I was also discontent with some of
the research and conceptual aspects of
the program. Traditional psychological
assessment techniques were inadequate to
measure many of the changes that were occurring and more emphasis should have been
placed on the school system as well as on
broader socioeconomic problems. It was
clear that many of the problems were shared
with other early-intervention projects.
I was undecided at the completion of the
intervention whether to write a general
description of the project or a critique
of these kinds of early intervention programs. The final result (Thomas, Chinsky,
& Aronson, 1973) was a combination of the
two and is probably one of the few research reports with its own attached critique.

A Behavioral Assessment of a Ward Environment

The behavioral assessment of a ward of institutionalized retarded children is one of two major projects with which I have been most recently involved. My principal coworkers are George Allen, another faculty member; Steven Veit, a graduate student; Wayne Dailey, Joan Harris, and nine other talented undergraduates. The director of the psychology department at the institution, Jack Thaw, is also an important member of the collaboration team. The goal of the project is to systematically observe, describe, and ultimately improve the interpersonal life of the retarded child.

The institution has a resident population of about 1500. The particular focus of our intervention is a ward having approximately 37 children between the ages of five and 15. They ranged from moderately to profoundly retarded and all are ambulatory. The staff includes 18 aides, 11 from the first shift and seven from the second. The average ratio of staff to patients is one to 12. Very few children are discharaged to the community although a few are sometimes transferred to another ward.

The project evolved from an attempt to implement a behavior modification program on this ward. Several undergraduates had begun training the children three or four hours a week but little change seemed to be occurring. The difficulty did not appear to be with the children; they made gains within the course of a session, but these were lost between training meetings.

I was especially attuned to this kind of problem because of my previous experience at Rochester State Hospital. It is futile to work with residents of an institution for a limited number of hours a week when they have to return to a custodial vacuum. Many of the improvements in behavior that are made in treatment are extinguished in the day-to-day environment of the ward.

We discontinued the behavior modification phase of the project and considered alternative courses of action. Rather than sever our contact with the institution, which now had a one-year history, we decided to develop a method of studying and improving the overall living environment for these children. We decided, in a sense, to try to reawaken another "Sleeping Dragon" (Rappaport, Chinsky, & Cowen, 1971).

There has been a great deal of anecdotal material about wards for retarded but, with few exceptions (e.g., Klaber, 1971), little systematic research. One of the problems has been the absence of a way of reliably and objectively describing this environment. We decided to develop a recording system to achieve this purpose. Our first step was a series of 24-hour observation sessions in which we noted all possible interactions on the ward.

We found that about 75 percent of the interactions were between aides and residents and decided to focus on these.

About six months were spent revising and testing before a method that was objective, reliable, and broad enough to encompass the major features of these interactions was designed.

The Interaction Recording System (IRS) measures several characteristics of aide-resident communications including: 1) affective tone--positive, negative, or neutral; and 2) the context in which these interactions occur--ward care, child care, formal training, and social-play. Ward care refers to routine activities such as cleaning the ward. Child care includes personal care involving the child's physical needs, such as putting on a child's shoes or getting him dressed for breakfast. Formal training is defined as teaching the child self-care skills. Social-play is scored when the child and aide are interacting in a personal way such as playing or talking, not in response to the child's physical needs. Also scored are 3) the initiator of the interaction--resident or aide; 4) the mode of interaction--physical and/or verbal; 5) whether or not the communication was a command; and 6) the response of the recipient--comply, ignore, or resist. In addition, such features as the time, room, and number of aides and residents present are noted. A manual was written for the IRS and we have found that the system can be learned in about six hours to 80 percent overall agreement by novice raters (Veit, 1973).

Students spent a good deal of time on the ward, both during the behavior modification program and while the IRS was

being modified. Many of the observers
and aides were on a first name basis after this year-and-a-half period. This
preparation allowed us to conduct our formal systematic observations with little
resistance on the part of the staff. Our
observations are, thus, probably more
representative of the actual ward environment than those that might have been obtained had we begun our recording abrupt-
ly as strangers. In fact, these observations would probably be impossible to
make under such circumstances.

Bias in the behavior of aides because
of our presence, had it occurred, would
have been in the favorable direction, i.e.
behavior would have appeared more positive
than it actually might have been. "Real"
conditions could only be worse than what
was observed. Considering how poor the
situation that we found was, the need for
improvement can only be underscored by
this possible bias.

Formal observations using the IRS
were first conducted for a 12-week period
in the spring of 1972. They covered the
two day shifts; night activity was not
recorded because our 24-hour investiga-
tions had shown that too few interactions
occurred at this time to warrant intensive recording. More than 20,000 15-se-
cond observations of aide-resident interactions were made during this period.

These observations have allowed us
to clearly describe the general nature of
the relationships between the children
and aides and have led to a number of interesting findings. For example, we found

that the average child on the ward received only 4.5 minutes of formal training a day. This amount differed greatly
for each individual child as aides spent
a disproportionate amount of time with
various residents (Dailey, Allen, Chinsky,
& Veit, in press). Subsequent sorting
techniques revealed that aides spend more
time with residents perceived as likeable
and attractive whereas less fortunate
children are virtually ignored. Another
study showed that outside volunteers tend
to more frequently visit the same more
fortunate residents.

Using the IRS we have also studied
specific influences such as room size and
the ratio of staff to patients. With regard to the latter, we have found that
the notion of staff/patient ratios is
more complicated than typically considered. There is a marked difference in the
quality of interactions between one aide
and nine children than between two aides
and eighteen children, although the ratio
is constant.

Another part of the study involves
the development of a method of using the
IRS with videotape recording of the ward.
We have also been studying the effect of
a remote-controlled videotape camera on
ward behavior (Spencer, Corcoran, Allen,
Chinsky, & Veit, 1974).

As part of our general observations,
a new aide, who started on the ward about
the same time we began using the IRS, was
tracked behaviorally over the course of a
12-week period. He decided to quit at the
end of this time and thus we had a beha-

vioral sample of his entire tenure as an
aide.   In a subsequent recorded interview, he told one of our undergraduates
that he decided to quit because he felt
he was being forced to conform to the
custodial routine. He told her that he
began by trying to be a friend to the
children and interact socially with them.
Over time, he became more ward oriented
and finally after several weeks he gave
up and changed his approach. Our independent behavioral observations confirmed
his reports and revealed the process of
institutionalization of his behavior including a sudden and dramatic decrease in
his social-play interactions (Allen, Chinsky, & Veit, 1974).

Observations were begun again in the
spring of 1973 to study the effect of an
inservice training program aimed at teaching aides behavior modification techniques.
An adaptation of the IRS was used to provide a comprehensive behavioral assessment
of the effect of this program on actual
ward behavior. This form of assessment is
especially important as we have found that
aides' responses on paper-and-pencil questionnaires, which have frequently been
used in the past to assess inservice training, have little to do with their actual
interactions on the ward.

A very important part of our project
involves providing feedback to the institution so that suggestions for improvements of environmental and interpersonal
conditions can be made. Such feedback was
for the benefit of both staff and residents and was not at the expense of specific individuals within the system. The

institution has been very supportive of
our work and many changes have been implemented or planned. Further research involving other wards is being formulated and
the collaborative relationship in a variety of forms is likely to be continued for
many years even as treatment practices improve and the institution becomes more
oriented to the community.

A Multilevel Intervention in an Elementary School

My association with a local school
system began about four years ago when I
provided WISC and WPPSI reports on some
of their students through a graduate class
in psychological testing. During this
time, I met guidance counselors, principals, many teachers, and the superintendent of schools. The previous year we had
attempted a small project in one of the
schools. This project, involving building
affective skills, was not successful but
served the wider purpose of increasing my
contact with the school and laying the
foundation for the development of a full-
scale intervention.

One of the graduate students had indicated an interest in primary prevention
involving the training of problem-solving
skills. Another wanted to conduct a companionship program with a high-risk population. A third was interested in working
with George Allen on a behavior modification program. It was decided to integrate
all three approaches simultaneously in an
attempt to encompass the full range of
mental health services to the school.

After a semester and a summer of preliminary negotiations with the principal
and several teachers, a complete program
was developed. Although the three projects were closely interrelated, each was
designed with its own subgoals, controls,
and evaluation strategies.

An informal contract detailing each
of the programs to be offered was presented to a meeting of the entire faculty in
the early fall of 1972. We estimated the
cost of services to be $5,000 at a mini-
mum but offered to do the project free in
return for the opportunity to evaluate it.
The exact time and tasks required of each
teacher for service and evaluation were
specified for the entire intervention.
The teachers and staff agreed to participate in the project and support it. An
outline of the intervention is presented
in Table 2.

The school consists of 19 third and
fourth grade classes and has a total of
about 480 students. The 19 classrooms
are divided into relatively independent
units of four or five classes each. Curricula for each unit are decided by the
teachers headed by a unit leader after
consultation with the principal.

Stephen Larcen (1973) was responsi-
ble for the primary prevention aspect of
the program and it was his original idea
to combine the three projects into one
large intervention. He worked with one
unit of four teachers, training them to
teach problem-solving skills in their
classes. Exercises were planned for two
half hours a week for about five months

following a workbook designed for the program. Children were given practice in divergent thinking, problem identification, and the generation and elaboration of solutions, as well as how to consider the outcomes of these solutions (D'Zurrilla & Goldfried, 1971). Problem-solving strategies were applied to real-life problems of the eight- to ten-year-old child. Several videotapes were made for the project to be used for modeling purposes. Preliminary results from paper-and-pencil measures as well as behavioral indices have shown the program to be markedly successful.

Howard Selinger (1973) developed a companionship program which operated during recess and lunch periods. The companions were 22 college students trained to work specifically with socially withdrawn children. Social withdrawal has been called a "non-behavior disorder" (O'Connor, 1969). These children are frequently overlooked in school yet many may develop more serious interpersonal difficulties later in life.

Children were selected on the basis of teacher referrals and behavioral observations during recess time. While playing with the children, companions used a variety of behavioral techniques aimed at improving their social skills and increasing their positive interactions with peers. Many of the children developed close and affectionate ties with their companions and improvements in behavior have been noted anecdotally and through systematic mid- and post-program behavioral observations.

The third level was directed by Jack Lochman (1973) who worked with six teachers in a series of nine workshops on behavior modification skills. Training included such things as targeting behavioral deficits, use of contingency contracting, selecting appropriate reinforcers, etc. In addition, each teacher was given the task of implementing a behavior-shaping program with one or two of the most disruptive or academically deficient students. Assessment has included the effect of such training on the specific children involved as well as changes in the participant teachers' classrooms. By contrasting these classrooms with those of the six control teachers, we are studying the radiating effect of the consultation process (Kelly, 1971).

The multilevel intervention, which has been described very briefly, required an extensive collaborative effort between the university and the school system. Besides two faculty members and three graduate students, more than 70 undergraduates were directly involved in the program. In addition, almost every teacher, special service staff member, and student in the elementary school participated in some way. We were quite interested in the impact of the program on the entire school system and investigated this area as well.

A follow-up project has been designed for the next year with plans for continued research, particularly in the area of problem solving. In accord with my views on successful community intervention, resources have been developed within the school to continue all three forms of service.

Contributions to Community Psychology

The nature of the projects described above defines, in many ways, my contribution to the community movement. In the first place, the projects demonstrate that meaningful research can be applied to social problems. This point will be discussed in more detail in the next section. In addition, this approach is being taught to graduate students directly involved in these programs as well as others in a graduate seminar that I teach. Thus, new professionals are being trained with an understanding of community problems and experience in community research.

Many undergraduates use the interventions as a testing ground for deciding whether to pursue a career in the field. Because of this background, some of the undergraduates choose to enter M.A. or Ph.D. programs in community or clinical psychology. Others may go into direct service roles at the B.A. level. These students have been well trained not only in behavior technology but also in thinking critically about assessment and new treatment approaches. For those students who don't stay in the field, these projects perform the functions of providing a personally meaningful experience in a community setting and acquainting them directly with some of the problems of our society.

The institution or community group is shown that it can work in a mutually beneficial and collaborative way with the university. Academic research in the past has too often had very little pay-off for the community and many groups feel that they have been exploited.

THE FUTURE OF COMMUNITY PSYCHOLOGY

This section will offer first a discussion of my personal plans and second some of my views on the future of the field. My personal interests first include a continuation of the type of community mental health interventions with which I have been engaged. I enjoy working with the collaborative intervention design and learning more of the subtleties of community research. One of my future goals is to innovate a program within a geriatric setting. Both environmental assessment and new treatment alternatives would be quite useful and applicable to this population.

Another area of interest involves working with students on systems level research. A possible training sequence might first include service work, perhaps on a ward or for a community agency. This would provide the student with the essential experience of feeling what it is like to be at the ground level of the setting, and directly acquaint him with its strengths and weaknesses. Based on this experience, the student could then investigate the structure of the system in which he was working, including studies of decision-making processes and sources of change in the institution or community.

A third area of interest is primary prevention programs using social problem-solving training. This approach has many advantages, particularly in schools. Because it teaches strategies of problem solving rather than any specific content, it is relatively value free. In a sense, it gives the individual the chance to choose what he considers his problem to be. Problem-solving training is also more specific in purpose and method than t-groups or other affect-building experiences and, thus, more amenable to a school curriculum.

The approach fosters self-competence, focusing on providing the individual with skills to help him solve his own problems. Many solutions, of course, would involve cooperation and learning how to interact with others in a positive and meaningful way. Another very important aspect of the approach is that it is a preventative strategy divorced from the notions of mental health or illness. It emphasizes building coping skills and can be taught to all children without possible stigma. Finally, the approach is researchable. Because it has benefit as a worthwhile ability in itself, it can be measured immediately after the intervention. Long-term favorable effects can be measured in subsequent follow-up studies.

Despite these positive attributes, two important cautions need to be considered. First, one would have to be careful not to generalize from this approach and blame the individual for the problem (Ryan, 1971). Second, the approach does not relinquish the need to make important

changes in our society so that more alternatives for problem solving are genuinely available to poor, ghetto children.

It would be easy to write a whole paper or, more likely, several volumes, on
the future of community psychology since
the field is so broad and intertwined with
the very essence of man in his environment. Short of that I will discuss a few
issues that I consider salient from my
vantage point.

First, it appears that "the honeymoon
is over." Initially any project under the
rubric of community psychology was valued
because it was new and offered an innovative approach to old problems. Most reports were descriptive and the ratio of
words to numbers was exceedingly high.
Despite the rhetoric and the hopes, however, the problems are still around and
in fact seem to be getting worse. A heal-
thy skepticism for community approaches
tends to be growing and there is an increasing need for more evaluative research.
Fortunately, I think community psychologists are beginning to meet this need. It
is no accident that two empirically-ori-
ented journals designed exclusively for
the community research worker have recently appeared. A few years ago, they
would both have probably gone out of
business.

Shifts in federal funding away from
graduate education will probably mean an
increase in community research. Graduate
students will have to work in applied settings to earn enough money to go to school,
and will probably do more research in

these locations. If such research does
increase, it will be a classical example
of the right thing for the wrong reasons.

The basic challenge confronting the
field today is the need to demonstrate
that theory and research can be meaning-
fully applied to social problems. Too
often in the past, researchers have had
to choose between sophisticated methodology and socially significant results.
We need to develop research strategies
and theories to study such areas as urban stress, overpopulation, drug use,
technological change, and the multitude
of other problems involving the effects
of the environment on man. We also need
to develop viable prevention programs to
reduce the ever-increasing number of social casualties. Community psychology
holds the unique link between systematic
research and social change. Certainly,
considering the vast problems of the late
twentieth century, such a convergence has
never been more necessary. To quote Fairweather (1972):

. . . an effective mechanism for social change requires the continuous
creation and evaluation of new models
for a given social problem, even where
a model has been found to be more beneficial than existing practices and
is in the process of being implemented.
It is this continuous and neverending
search for new physical and social innovations to solve particular human
problems that can provide society with
workable and predictable inventions
that can improve the quality of life.
Anything less might deny future gene-

rations a democratic society and a
livable environment /p. 30/.

ACKNOWLEDGMENTS

Collaborative research, by definition, could not be done within the help
of many people. Only some of them are
mentioned by name in the text of this paper. I am especially indebted to Dr.
Julian Rappaport and Dr. Emory L. Cowen
for their initial and continued support.
Dr. Julian Rotter and my other colleagues
at the Psychology Department of the University of Connecticut have provided the
scholarly and creative atmosphere necessary for my work. Dr. George Allen has
been an invaluable partner in my later research.

Research described in the paper has
been funded in part by the Psychology Departments of the University of Rochester
and the University of Connecticut; the
Maurice Falk Medical Fund; the Connecticut
Department of Mental Health, Division of
Community Services; the University of Connecticut Research Foundation; and NSF
Grant GJ-9 to the University of Connecticut Computer Center. Special thanks are
due to Ms. Elizabeth Caine for her translation and typing of the original cassette
tape. This paper is dedicated to my personal collaborator, Mariann.

REFERENCES

Albee, G. W. The relation of conceptual
    models to the manpower problem. In E.

L. Cowen, E. A. Gardner, & M. Zax (Eds.) Emergent approaches to mental health problems. New York: Appleton, 1967. Pp. 63-73.

Allen, G. J., Chinsky, J. M., & Veit, S. W. Pressures toward institutionalization within the aide culture: A behavioral-analytic case study. Journal of Community Psychology, 1974, 2, 67-70.

Ansama, J. W., Jr. The effects of modeling, expectancy, and intimacy level on self-disclosing behavior. Unpublished masters study, University of Connecticut, 1974.

Bambrough, B. An investigation of the construct of accurate empathy. Unpublished masters study, University of Connecticut, 1973.

Chinsky, J. M. Nonprofessionals in a mental hospital: A study of the college student volunteer. Unpublished doctoral dissertation, University of Rochester, 1968.

Cowen, E. L. Emergent approaches to mental health problems: An overview and directions for future work. In E. L. Cowen, E. A. Gardner, & M. Zax (Eds.) Emergent approaches to mental health problems. New York: Appleton, 1967. Pp. 389-455.

Cowen, E. L., Chinsky, J. M., & Rappaport, J. Un undergraduate practicum in community mental health. Community Mental Health Journal, 1970, 6, 91-100.

Dailey, W. F., Allen, G. J., Chinsky, J. M., & Veit, S. W. Relationships between attendant behavior and attitudes toward institutionalized retarded children. American Journal of Mental Deficiency, in press.

D'Augelli, A. R., & Chinsky, J. M. Interpersonal skills and pretraining: Implications for the use of group procedures for interpersonal learning and for the selection of nonprofessional mental health workers. Journal of Consulting and Clinical Psychology, in press.

D'Augelli, A. R., Chinsky, J. M., & Getter, H. The effect of group composition and duration on sensitivity training. Small Group Studies, in press.

D'Zurilla, T. J., & Goldfried, M. R. Problem solving and behavior modification. Journal of Abnormal Psychology, 1971, 78, 107-126.

Fairweather, G. W. Social change: The challenge to survival. Morristown, N. J.: General Learning Press, 1972.

Golann, S. E. Community psychology and mental health: An analysis of strategies and a survey of training. In I. Iscoe & C. D. Spielberger (Eds.) Community psychology: Perspectives in training and research. New York: Appleton, 1970. Pp. 33-57.

Goodman, G. Companionship therapy. San Francisco: Jossey-Bass, 1972.

Kelly, J. G. Antidotes for arrogance:

Training for community psychology. _American Psychologist_, 1970, 25, 524-531.

Kelly, J. G. The quest for valid preventive interventions. In G. Rosenblum (Ed.) _Issues in community psychology and preventive mental health_. New York: Behavioral Publications, 1971. Pp. 109-139.

Kiesler, D. J. Some myths of psychotherapy research and the search for paradigm. _Psychological Bulletin_, 1966, 65, 110-136.

Klaber, M. M. _Retardates in residences: A study of institutions_. West Hartford, Conn.: University of Hartford Press, 1969.

Larcen, S. W. Training in social problem solving: A preventive intervention in the school. Unpublished masters study, University of Connecticut, 1973.

Lochman, J. E. Consultation to elementary school teachers: A behavior modification workshop. Unpublished masters study, University of Connecticut, 1973.

O'Conner, R. D. Modeling treatment of non-behavior disorders. Paper presented at meeting of the Midwestern Psychological Association, Chicago, May, 1969.

Poser, E. G. The effects of therapist training on group therapeutic outcome. _Journal of Consulting Psychology_, 1966, 30, 283-289.

Rappaport, J. Nonprofessionals in a mental hospital: College students as group leaders with chronic patients. Unpublished doctoral dissertation. University of Rochester, 1968.

Rappaport, J., Chinsky, J. M., & Cowen, E. L. Innovations in helping chronic patients: College students in a mental institution. New York: Academic Press, 1971.

Rotter, J. B. The future of clinical psychology. Journal of Consulting and Clinical Psychology, 1973, 40, 313-321.

Ryan, W. Blaming the victim. New York: Pantheon, 1971.

Schofield, W. Psychotherapy: The purchase of friendship. Englewood Cliffs, N.J.: Prentice-Hall, 1964.

Selinger, H. V. A behaviorally oriented companionship program for socially deficient children. Unpublished masters study, University of Connecticut, 1973.

Spencer, F. W., Corcoran, C. A., Allen, G. W., Chinsky, J. M., & Veit, S. W. Reliability and reactivity of the videotape technique on a ward for retarded children. Journal of Community Psychology, 1974, 2, 71-74.

Thomas, P. H., Chinsky, J. M., & Aronson, C. F. A preschool educational program with Puerto Rican children: Implications as a community intervention. Journal of Community Psychology, 1973, 1, 18-22.

Truax, C. B., & Carkhuff, R. R.   Toward
    effective counseling and psychotherapy:
    Training and practice.   Chicago: Aldine,
    1967.

Veit, S. W.   A method for investigating
    interactions between institutionalized
    retardates and their aides.   Unpublished
    masters study, University of Connecti-
    cut, 1973.

Whithorn, J. C., & Betz, B. J.   A study
    of psychotherapeutic relationships be-
    tween physicians and schizophrenic pa-
    tients.   American Journal of Psychiatry,
    1954, 111, 321-331.

3. COMMUNITY PSYCHOLOGY AND MENTAL
HEALTH ADMINISTRATION: FROM THE
FRYING PAN INTO THE FIRE

Gershen Rosenblum

When I was invited to participate in
this symposium it was suggested that I
1) give a brief autobiographical sketch
as a case example of the evolution of a
"community psychologist," and 2) define
my current role as a regional mental
health administrator for the Massachusetts Department of Mental Health. To
the best of my ability this is what I
will now attempt to do.

FROM CLINICAL PSYCHOLOGY TO COMMUNITY PSYCHOLOGY IN ONE DIFFICULT LESSON

My professional career as a traditional clinical psychologist began when
I was accepted to the clinical psychology
doctoral program at Boston University in
the late 1940's. After placements and
internships at the Massachusetts General
Hospital, Boston State Hospital, Judge
Baker Guidance Clinic, and James Jackson
Putnam Children's Center in Boston, I
finally received my doctorate and pro-

ceeded to work for the next seven years
at mental health clinics in the Greater
Boston area as a traditional psychologist
providing individual and group psychotherapy, psychological testing, and engaging
in research with cleft palate and hospi-
talized children. In early 1960, I accepted a position as a chief psychologist
at the South Shore Mental Health Center in
Quincy, Massachusetts, where a quiet re-
volution in the provision of community
mental health services was taking place.
What was occurring at this clinic which I
found exciting was the conscious decision
of one key person there to try to provide
consultation services to the schools,
clergy, courts, and police in the South
Shore area as an alternative to the bur-
densome waiting list which was increasing
weekly as the inadequate numbers of clinic personnel found themselves unequal to
the task of evaluating and treating the
large numbers of persons who were referred for treatment. It was hoped that the
numbers of referrals could be reduced if
the major sources of those referrals--
the schools, clergy, courts, and police
--were helped in their role of caregivers
to the community. Thus, a couple of psychologists were assigned the task of providing case consultation to several community agencies. It was a difficult process
to educate the community groups in the
appropriate way of utilizing consultation;
namely, as one professional assisting another to sharpen his skills rather than
adopting a "doctor-patient" transference
relationship as some consultees were wont
to do.

At about the same time, Dr. Gerald Caplan of the Harvard School of Public Health was developing his concepts of mental health consultation and offered a course on this subject to selected Department of Mental Health employees. Not knowing what mental health consultation was, I decided to attend his lectures for an academic year; during the same period I was accompanying a colleague from the clinic into the schools of a South Shore community. It was from this modest beginning over a decade ago that I began to be aware of the limitations of the traditional psychological role. Concurrently, I became excited by the possibility that there might be other ways of helping people rather than waiting for them to come to a mental health clinic with a debilitating emotional disorder and undergoing individual or group psychotherapy. While still functioning, for the most part, as a traditional psychologist I found myself increasingly involved in community mental health activities. As I recall, at that time we did not utilize terms like "community mental health" or "community psychology." Instead, we talked about "community consultation," although that phrase was never succinctly defined.

A number of serendipitous events occurred during the next five to six years which propelled me into the vanguard of the community psychology movement and changed my whole perspective of how psychologists can best "help" people function optimally. The first event took place in the summer of 1962 when Dr. Caplan, who had just concluded an agreement with the Psychology Department at Duke University

to instruct two graduate students for
twelve weeks in the principles of mental
health consultation, asked the South Shore
Mental Health Clinic to find community
placements for these students two days a
week and to assume supervisory responsibility
over their community assignments. We accepted the challenge and were immediately
faced with the task of finding appropriate
community settings for them during the
summer. (Our major source of community
placements were the schools and they, of
course, were closed down during this period.) We finally decided to work out arrangements for these students with the
Quincy Welfare Department where they were
assigned the task of setting up educational programs and discussion groups
to aid welfare mothers who were encountering difficulties with their children. The
evaluations by the students at the end of
the summer spoke so highly of their community experience in Quincy that the following spring the officials at Duke University by-passed the Harvard School of
Public Health completely and negotiated
directly with the South Shore Clinic for a
full-time summer community experience for
two of their graduate students. This arrangement continued to the mutual advantage of both Duke and South Shore for the
next several summers. It was during this
period that considerable thought was given
to ways whereby the community could be
served more effectively by mental health
professionals.

The Boston Conference on the Education of
Psychologists for Community Mental Health

It was not until 1965 that I began to

grasp fully what "community psychology"
was or could be. Dr. Joseph Spiesman,
who at that time was Chief of the Psychology Training Program at the National Institute for Mental Health, had invited
John Glidewell of the Social Science Research Unit at Washington University in
St. Louis to convene a conference dealing with the education and training of
psychologists in community mental health.
Dr. Glidewell, due to other commitments,
was unable to accept and suggested that
Dr. Spiesman call us at South Shore. He
followed through on this suggestion and
we found ourselves being asked to organize a conference in the Greater Boston
area together with one of the Boston area
universities. We thought immediately of
Boston University because of the work
which Dr. Donald Klein of the Boston University Human Relations Laboratory was
doing in facilitating "helping relationships" between community caregivers and
consumers in need. And so we invited Dr.
Klein and Dr. Chester Bennett, the chair-
man of the Clinical Psychology program at
Boston University, to sit down with three
of us from South Shore--Saul Cooper,
Leonard Nassol, and me--and help plan a
three-and-one-half day conference on the
education of psychologists in community
mental health (which we eventually held
at Swampscott, a small scenic seacoast
town north of Boston). It was this conference that opened up new vistas for me
in formulating and conceiving the parameters of community psychology.

Many of the psychologists' names
which were proposed for inclusion in this
conference were new to me. Likewise, I

presented some names which were unknown
to the others. After much discussion of
the backgrounds and potential contributions which might be made by various individuals, we finally settled on 39 persons
(including the five members of the conference committee, a conference coordinator,
and six observers from NIMH). We managed
to get a very interesting and broad as-
sortment of participants with diverse experiences and perceptions of the problem.
As we began the task of defining the mandate of the conference--issues related
to the training of psychologists in community mental health--it became apparent
to the majority of us that community mental health was only a portion or a subspecialty of a larger concept which we
ultimately labeled as community psychology. New ideas and insights were generated
by various psychologists functioning in
unorthodox settings or with unusual backgrounds, such as Arthur Pearl, who was
heavily involved in providing new mental
health programs for the poor; Bob Reiff,
a former labor union organizer who was
developing the concept of the indigenous
nonprofessional; Ija Korner, who had spent
six months sitting in the office of the
Governor of Utah in order to ascertain the
psychological impact on the community of
political decision-making; Jim Kelly, who
was studying the relationship between ecology and mental health; and Mort Brown,
who was the assistant to the Illinois Commissioner of Mental Health. We had a gathering of very unusual and articulate people and it was an extremely productive
conference. I've been to many conferences
before and since, but I can't recall any
other that generated as many ideas during

the meetings or stimulated as many activities and programs subsequent to the
conference as this one (e.g., Division 27
--Division of Community Psychology--of
A.P.A., the Community Mental Health Journal, the mushrooming of university training programs in community pscyhology and
community mental health, etc.). The terms
"community psychology" and "participant-
conceptualizer" which were coined during
the conference proceedings reflected the
broadening definition of the community
mental health psychologist's role and the
unique contribution which, by virtue of
his educational background and training,
he could add to the planned change process in the community. At the same time
there emerged an increasing realization
that to become a true community psychologist one had to become conversant with
subject matters heretofore quite alien
to the traditional fields of knowledge to
which the clinical psychology student was
exposed--generally, the areas of psycho-
diagnosis, therapy, and research. Knowledge of such areas as community organization, urban planning, economics, law enforcement, public health, ecology, and
epidemiology were suggested by several
participants as necessary if the community psychologist were to function effectively in the community. Others began
to question the relationship of these diverse subject areas to psychology. The
question was raised as to whether a new
discipline was being advocated which had
only peripheral ties to psychology. They
asked, "Why do we believe that psychologists are able to carry out this community role any more effectively (or even
as effectively) as, for example, a social

worker, or a public health nurse, or a
cultural anthropologist, or a sociolo-
gist?" The questions which were posed
during that memorable conference are still
being debated and explored to the present
day in an attempt to define the nature and
parameters of this emerging specialized
area of community services.

TRAINING IN COMMUNITY PSYCHOLOGY
AND COMMUNITY MENTAL HEALTH

The insights which were gleaned from
the Boston Conference led to a determination to train budding psychologists in
community mental health at South Shore
Clinic (and in community psychology as
well, to the extent that it was possible
within the confines of a community mental health setting). In 1965, the clinic received four summer stipends from
NIMH for training clinical psychology students in the art of community psychology.
We began with a two-summer program but
this arrangement led to commitment problems and interfered with dissertation research so that we subsequently modified
it to an intensive three-month internship
during the course of one summer. Students
were placed in numerous settings in the
community--community action agencies, law
enforcement agencies, prison clinics,
Headstart classes, summer camps, etc.--
under close supervision. They were
taught skills in mental health consultation, community organization, social advocacy, anticipatory guidance, and political
science. They learned how to appraise the
problems of an individual which had been
shaped, influenced, or made inevitable by

the community in which he was rooted, as
well as the problems of the community which
helped shape the destinies of the individuals who lived within its confines. The
students were at times victorious, frustrated, exhilarated, exhausted, but never
bored! By 1967, six or seven universities
(Duke U., U. of Florida, U. of Colorado,
U. of Nebraska, Florida State U., U. of
Texas, Vanderbilt U.) were vying to place
summer students at South Shore. Students
were coming with a diversity of backgrounds
and unique experiences in working within
their local communities. While we were
teaching them what we knew, we were simultaneously absorbing fresh bright ideas
from our interns. Many have subsequently
gone forth as a second generation of community psychologists and are making names
for themselves in academic and community
settings around the country.

MENTAL HEALTH ADMINISTRATION, OR "IF YOU CAN'T STAND THE HEAT, GET THE HELL OUT OF THE KITCHEN"

In November of 1967, I became a regional mental health administrator for the
Massachusetts Department of Mental Health.
While it was only six years ago it seems
like half a lifetime. Mental health administration in Massachusetts, which heretofore had been confined to boarded psychiatrists and which had proceeded at a
leisurely pace, was finally made available to psychologists (and later on to a
wide variety of mental health and retardation professionals) as a result of a re-
organization of the Massachusetts Department of Mental Health.

Try to visualize the mental health
scene in the Commonwealth of Massachusetts
in the Spring and Summer of 1967. The
legislature had just reluctantly passed
an act reorganizing the Commonwealth into
seven mental health regions (which were
further subdivided into 39 areas). By
strenuous lobbying efforts a coalition
of interested citizen groups and psychologists were successful (by a one-vote
margin) in including A.B.P.P. psychologists as well as psychiatrists as eligible to fill all the newly created key
administrative posts in the Department of
Mental Health (with the exception of two
--the Commissioner and Deputy Commissioner
of Mental Health). The positions included
five assistant commissioners, seven regional mental health administrators, seven
regional mental retardation administrators,
and seven regional legal medicine direc-
tors--26 administrative positions in all.

The state psychiatric and medical societies were especially furious at the
state-employed psychologists who had lob-
bied so hard to expand the qualifications
for the administrative posts and these societies were united in their efforts to
dissuade the Commissioner of Mental Health
from filling the positions with other than
psychiatrists. The Commissioner was under
a great deal of pressure to accede to
these demands. He had lived and worked
in Massachusetts all his life; he was an
active member in the psychiatric community; many of the persons who were im-
portuning him were close colleagues and
might well consider him a "traitor" should
he break ranks with their determinantion
to exclude nonmedical candidates from con-

sideration for the administrative jobs.
On the other side of the coin, few qualified psychiatrists were actively seeking the newly created posts; the pay was
not especially high in relation to the
salaries which psychiatrists could earn
in private practice; and many psychiatrists did not find the demanding and often frustrating role of a mental health
administrator to be their "cup of tea."
So, the weeks went by, only a few of the
administrative positions were filled (by
psychiatrists), and the Massachusetts
Association for Mental Health which had
fought so hard for the passage of the re-
organization act was beginning to criti-
cize the Commissioner for not moving more
quickly in carrying out the mandate of
the new law.

It was in this climate that I decided
to make my move to become the first nonmedical regional mental health administrator in the Commonwealth. For me it seemed
a natural progression in my career from a
clinical-community chief psychologist of
a well established community mental health
clinic (the position of Director of a Mental Health Clinic at that time was not
open to nonmedical professionals) to the
administrative regional head of several
clinics and institutions. In my prior
role I had only limited means to implement new ideas or to influence others in
moving in new directions. In the new position I felt that I would be able to expand my role as a "participant-conceptu-
alizer" and have a more significant impact
in generating change. Besides, I felt
that I was as well qualified as my psychiatric colleagues to fill such a posi-

tion and I was challenged by the prospect of breaking new ground in the as yet undefined role of a regional mental health administrator. Also, if I could pave the way as the first nonmedical mental health administrator in the Commonwealth, it would be easier for others to follow.

Thus, I formally applied for the position of mental health administrator of Region V and several weeks passed by without any word from the Commissioner. In the meantime, the psychiatric directors of mental health facilities in Region V began to hold regular meetings for the purpose of recruiting a psychiatrist for the regional administrator position who would be acceptable to them and whom they could then recommend to the Commissioner. As the meetings dragged on week after week, it became apparent that they were unable to agree on any psychiatric candidate willing to accept the position. The superintendents of the state institutions were unwilling to accept a psychiatrist who was identified with the community clinics; the clinic directors were suspicious of the inbred ideas of those institution-based psychiatrists who indicated their availability. Their mutual fears that a particular facility would be short-changed by a psychiatric administrator favoring a differing philosophy of mental health care or treatment led inevitably to an impasse.

It was at about this time that I arranged for a personal interview with the Commissioner. As President of the Massachusetts Psychological Association, I had recently had some dealings with him regarding the role of psychologists in the

mental health system in Massachusetts;
thus, he knew me slightly. During the
interview he was very cordial but indicated that the time was not ripe for him
to appoint a nonmedical person to the regional administrator's position. Naturally, I was disappointed; however, since he
had not turned me down but had merely de-
ferred his decision, I decided to take a
bold step and meet with the regional group
of psychiatrists who were still trying to
come up with a candidate they could all
agree on. My interview with this group
was reminiscent of the oral examination
of my doctoral dissertation. After asking
me a number of relevant and irrelevant
questions (such as, was I pro psychology?)
they asked me to leave the room while they
deliberated among themselves. They must
have found me less threatening than they
had at first imagined (or else they were
thoroughly frustrated in their quest for
an acceptable psychiatrist) for after 15
minutes I was summoned back to the room
and informed that they, as a group, found
me to be an acceptable candidate for the
position and would so notify the Commissioner. (The next day when the Commissioner received their letter he immediately telephoned me and said, "Gersh,
you've proven to me that you're capable
of being a mental health administrator--
the job's yours.") Was it only six years
ago? In six short years the opportunities
for nonmedical professionals to climb the
mental health ladder have increased significantly. First, the qualifications
have been broadened to include doctoral
mental health professionals from a diversity of disciplines and backgrounds. Second, the range of positions for which

this group is now eligible includes the
positions of Commissioner of Mental Health,
Superintendent of State Hospitals and
State Schools, Director of Mental Health
Centers and Court Clinics, Chiefs of units
in State Hospitals and Schools, and, in
fact, virtually every administrative position in the Department.

The breech in the wall which I helped
institute in 1967 has resulted in a veri-
table flood of mental health professionals
of diverse disciplines and backgrounds oc-
cupying important administrative posts at
the central, regional, and area levels
within the mental health system. The major criterion today is the best qualified
person regardless of his degree.

Upon being granted my desire to become a mental health administrator, I
moved into a job which was brand new,
untested, and ill-defined. But that very
ambiguity made it possible to hew and
shape a meaningful role for the regional
administrator without becoming bogged down
in a morass of tradition. The job was being defined in the process of performing
it day to day. My orientation was in the
direction of developing broad-based community mental health centers while, at
the same time, attempting to nudge the
institutions into a more rehabilitative
and community-oriented stance. The process of change is always a slow one; resistance to change, which is inevitable,
only yields slowly and reluctantly. This
has to be recognized and coped with. In
bringing about administrative and organizational change one has to think in terms
of months and years rather than days and

weeks. (An administrative colleague of
mine in another state, recognizing the
agonizingly slow progress of change, coined
a "law" which states: "It always takes
longer than it takes.") It requires a
high level of frustration tolerance and
gratification delay. It means having to
grapple with bureaucratic ineptitude and
red tape, irrational directives and, worst
of all, no key official willing to make
decisions during periods of crisis. I
have often said that the easiest part of
my job is planning programs to meet the
unmet mental health and retardation needs
in the region; the hardest part is obtaining the funds and resources to implement
the plans. Trying to persuade a vast
bureaucratic structure to be responsive
to regional needs is where most of my energy is expended, often with minimal results. It's like trying to push a huge
boulder uphill--a tremendous amount of effort is utilized for each miniscule movement. And you can't afford to relax for
a moment or you'll be crushed flat. While
movement appears imperceptible from day
to day, in looking back over the past several years, it is pleasantly evident that
considerable progress in the quest of my
goals has been achieved; at the same time,
in peering ahead it is painfully evident
that there remains much still to be done.
I guess it is inevitable that one of the
occupational hazards of administrators is
the constant struggle with crises and
frustrations and the slow pace of progress.
It is helpful to retain a sense of humor
and a philosophical acceptance of the
realities of the job if one is to survive
in the long run. (Administrators are fond
of quoting slogans to this effect--viz.

"illegitimi non carburundum" or "don't
let the ba---rds wear you down"; "If you
can't stand the heat, get the Hell out of
the kitchen"; "administrators don't win
popularity contests"; etc.)

MENTAL HEALTH ADMINISTRATIVE ROLES

How has the role of the regional administrator become defined during the last
six years? What opportunities are available to assist him in doing his job effectively? What restrictions are placed
upon him which limit his ability to function? There are at least seventeen dis-
tinguishable roles which I have had to
assume in the course of carrying out my
duties. These are not necessarily dis-
crete roles, they overlap. However, they
will convey the kinds of knowledge which
I had to acquire in order to fulfill the
responsibilities of the job. Many of
these skills were acquired in situ over the
years in order to deal effectively with
issues as they arose.

a) Planner

The first and one of the most important roles is that of mental health
planner. This is a function in which the
administrator first has to assess the unmet needs of the community and the available resources, and then begin to plan
how to utilize the existing resources
more efficiently, how to develop new resources, and how to establish meaningful
priorities. This is not always as easy
as it seems. Often we are not able to
determine exactly what the needs of a com-

munity are (such as the need for specific
alcohol and drug programs) because reliable statistical data are hard to obtain;
often we cannot accurately assess the
available resources in the area because
we have narrow conceptions as to what a
community resource consists of. There
are numerous groups and agencies in every
community which could be utilized as potential mental health resources if we
would enlist their support and enhance
their contribution to the promotion of
better community mental health through
mental health consultation techniques.
I'm referring to such groups as visiting
nurses associations, police departments,
clergy, school personnel, YMCA's and YWCA's,
lawyers, pediatricians, service organizations (Lion's, Rotary, Jr. C. of C.'s,
etc.), and numerous organized community
groups who can be very effective in providing help if they receive support and back-
up assistance.

With respect to assessing needs in a
community, it is useful to apply criteria
based on public health concepts of primary, secondary, and tertiary prevention.[1]

---

[1]Primary prevention refers to the
prevention of disease (or disorders) before it affects a given population (co-
hort) or numerous population groups. Secondary prevention refers to the contain-
ment of disease (or disorders) shortly after it appears and before it becomes more
severe or spreads to other groups. Tertiary prevention refers to rehabilitation
of persons who have been affected by a debilitating disease (or disorder) in order

What kinds of programs can be developed
to anticipate problems which are likely
to occur in a population at risk and to
help forestall their occurrence? What
kind of programs can be developed to identify incipient problems and prevent them
from becoming more disabling? Finally,
what programs can be developed to rehabi-
litate individuals who have already suc-
cumbed to a severe emotional or mental
disorder? Once programs have been con-
ceived, they have to be measured against
political and economic realities before
they can be instituted. For example, is
the community ready to accept a program
within its midst, such as a community
residence for post-hospitalized patients?
Are funds available to establish such a
program; if not, what are the chances of
obtaining local, state, or federal financial support? If program development or
expansion is determined to be feasible,
how are the priorities established? How
does one measure the importance of one set
of unmet needs against another? These are
difficult decisions which an administrator
is constantly required to make. If he is
to make good decisions he would be wise
to seek help and advice from the citizens
in the community as well as professional
practitioners working there. First, he
gets the key people and groups in the community to articulate their needs as they
perceive them. Second, he relies upon
them to help establish priorities for that

---

to restore them, as much as possible, to
their prior state of health (or adjustment).

area for he realizes that the establishment of priorities should be undertaken
in large measure by consumers and not primarily by professionals who are sitting
in a faraway regional or state office deciding solely what programs would be most
worthwhile for a particular area. One of
the main functions of an administrator is
to listen to the community, provide some
input into the decision-making process,
and try to find a constructive balance
between the citizens' wishes and the administrator's professional knowledge and
understanding of the community. A question which is frequently asked is: Who
is the community? Actually, the community (for our purposes) consists of con-
geries of interest groups who are concerned about the provision (or lack of
provision) of certain services which they
hope will improve the "quality of life"
for themselves, their relatives, their
neighbors, and their friends. In the
field of mental health and retardation we
identify such groups as associations for
the mentally ill and the retarded; associations concerned with the alcoholic, the
drug-dependent person, the delinquent and
adult offender, the compulsive gambler,
etc.; special interest groups dealing with
populations at risk such as parents without partners; associations for retired
persons and the elderly, for the deaf and
blind, for children with learning disabilities and perceptual handicaps, etc.
Also included are citizen groups such as
the Area Boards who represent various seg-
ments of the community--business, labor,
education, religion, medicine, law, mi-
norities, youth, elderly, social service,
nursing, law enforcement, politicians,

etc.   These groups are either involved
personally with persons in distress or
know of others who require services and
programs which are lacking.   Their interest is to attempt to improve the quality of
life of the citizens in their area.   It's
important to listen to the voices of these
diverse citizen groups, recognizing at the
same time that many have their own biases
and special positions which they espouse.
The administrator then attempts to establish a hierarchy of needs for each area
based on his best assessment of the many
inputs which reach his ear.

The following is an example of how
community input can result in the development of an urgently needed service.   In
the South Shore area (south of Boston),
the mental health clinic has provided a
variety of outpatient services to children
and adults for over twenty years and it is
regarded as a highly reputable community
mental health facility.   However, it has
operated on a nine to five basis from Mon-
day to Friday with no coverage for psychiatric emergencies during the evenings and
weekends.   A number of groups in the community began a year or so ago to make
their wishes known to the clinic director
and the regional administrative director
about the need for such an emergency services.   Through their efforts the clinic
has now established an emergency telephone
service that provides the South Shore community with 24-hour coverage seven days a
week.   While the results in this case are
laudable a word of caution must be inject-
ed at this point.   Not all of the programs
or services requested by a segment of the
community can or should be considered as

high-priority items. The task of the administrator is to weigh the relative needs
of a particular community request for services with others being generated by different (or similar) community groups in
the area. He must also attempt to educate
the community to view local community mental health needs within an area-wide context rather than as a grouping of several
unrelated needs. Mere residence in a community doesn't automatically qualify a
person as an "expert" in assessing the
community's several needs. An individual
who may be concerned and knowledgeable
about the needs of the retarded may be
disinterested or ignorant about the equally important needs of the alcoholic or the
elderly. It is not only the responsibility of the mental health administrator
to coordinate planning efforts for an area
or region but also to ensure that the
needs of the various chronological seg-
ments of the community receive considera-
tion in the planning process (infants,
children, adolescents, adults, and elderly) as well as the varied populations at
risk (mentally ill, mentally retarded,
drug dependent, alcoholic, juvenile delinquent, adult offender, children with
learning disabilities, etc.). Planning
includes the ten services formulated by
the National Institute of Mental Health.
Five are considered essential services:
outpatient, inpatient, intermediate care,
emergency, and consultation and education.
The remaining five are recommended: diagnostic, rehabilitative, precare and after-
care, training, and research and evaluation.

b) Educator

A second role of the mental health
administrator is that of educator. The
educator role is particularly vital in
this era of citizen involvement and participation in the mental health planning
process. If citizens are to make meaningful decisions regarding the mental
health requirements of their community
they must learn how to assess needs effectively and how to communicate their
findings to other citizens, to mental
health professionals, and to local and
State legislators. It is important to
distinguish "educating" for "propagandiz-
ing"; the former pertains to the dissemination of essential information which
the community needs in order to make intelligent decisions, the latter implies
an attempt to convince the citizens of
the professionals' point of view. Education can take place at area board meetings, at regional advisory council meetings, at seminars and workshops, and on
the telephone or in person with citizens
during periods of crisis. Finally, the
educator role may include the training of
mental health administrators and teaching
at a local university in the areas of
community psychology and/or mental health
administration.

c) Organizer and Grant Writer

In addition to the planning role, the
mental health administrator is often called upon to help organize the plans into
workable programs (including personnel
needed, budget, etc.) and to assist in
writing grant proposals seeking funds to

implement the planned programs. In the
past, until the Nixon Administration cut
off funds authorized under the Community
Mental Health Centers Act of 1963, administrators frequently participated with
local area groups in writing and defending
construction-grant proposals and staffing-
grant proposals for comprehensive community mental health centers. Currently,
they assist in the drafting of program
proposals to be funded under Federal Title 4A (social services for the poor) or
under Title 314(d) (comprehensive mental
health planning).

d) Mental Health Consultant

The mental health administrator frequently receives calls from local organizations who either wish help in resolving
internal organizational struggles or who
would like assistance in improving their
effectiveness. Also, mental health institutions will turn to administrators
for advice and consultation when they are
facing problems or crises which threaten
to interrupt their functioning. Some background and experience in organizational
crisis intervention is useful in these instances.

e) Communicator

While the communicator role is related to that of educator, its primary purpose is to make readily available to all
interested parties materials and information about current happenings and recent
changes which may affect the decision-making process. To get meaningful interaction between the citizens and profession-

als it is important to communicate the
latest developments quickly and accurately. For example, you can't assume that if
you telephone the presidents of the area
boards about an important piece of information that all 21 members of each area
board will hear about it (or, if they do,
that the message will be transmitted accurately and without distortion). How
then does one communicate effectively?
As a regional administrator I've developed several channels through which I can
pass on useful information to several
groups of people in the region. One is
a regional newsletter which is mailed out
monthly to about 500 persons including
area board members, mental health and retardation associations, facility heads,
politicians, and others. The voluminous
amount of mail which daily arrives at my
desk is sorted and items of relevance and
importance are marked for inclusion in the
newsletter. The newsletter is kept brief
and succinct and is not meant to be a
folksy, breezy newspaper. It serves to
inform, to educate, and to solicit help
in times of crises. When controversial
items are published we are sure to get a
number of phone calls asking for more information or offering help. We know, thus,
that it is read widely and the information
therein is utilized by its readers.

Another communication device is the
regional annual report. This report of
60-70 pages includes the mental health and
retardation activities which have taken
place in the region during the current
year and plans for the immediate future.
Statistics are presented, budgets are
itemized, and proposed programs of need

are listed in priority order.

Third is a regional Directory of Human Services which is published biannually and distributed widely. The latest edition consists of 178 pages and includes listings of the following human services: general health services, mental health services, mental retardation services, alcoholism services, drug abuse services, rehabilitation services, and community social services (adoption, aged, antipoverty agencies, community centers, employment, family counseling, housing authorities, social security, unwed mother's homes, welfare, youth services, nursery schools). A free copy is sent to every school system, church, police station, library, social service agency, community center, town and city office, court, and mental health facility in the region. It assists caregivers in the community to refer persons with whom they come into contact to appropriate resources. Finally, scheduled meetings are held with facility directors, with area office directors, with regional advisory council members, and with mental health association directors. All this effort is only a start towards fully effective communication. I am constantly seeking ways to improve the communication process.

f) <u>Lobbyist</u>

The lobbying role is an important one for effective mental health administration. Several years ago after I had spent two solid days at the State House garnering support for several new programs in my region which were up for debate before the

legislature, one of my psychological colleagues expressed dismay that I would be
utilizing my professional talents as a
lobbyist (which he evidently considered
to be a very demeaning job). What he
failed to realize was that lobbying efforts, in the constructive sense of the
word, are essential in convincing authorities to fund vitally needed programs. If
one works for a government agency the
funding authority is the legislature--
thus, interpreting one's programs to legislators is necessary if they are to be
fully informed of the nature of the requests before them. Lobbying is not really a dirty word--many legislators welcome
any information which will help them make
intelligent decisions; that doesn't necessarily mean that they will vote in your
favor all the time. It's important to
know the names of all the legislators in
the region and to meet as many of them as
possible. Whenever legislators call for
information or to request a favor, I try
to do whatever I can without breeching
ethics or undermining the Department's
established process for dealing with patients or programs; in turn, I feel comfortable in calling these same legislators
to help me advance my programs through the
governmental bureaucracy when they get
bogged down. If lobbying and political
contact are transacted within ethical
bounds, the public is the ultimate gainer.

g) Architectural Consultant

A somewhat different role for the administrator is that of architectural consultant. In the process of setting up
comprehensive community mental health cen-

ter programs it behooves the mental health
administrator to be conversant with architectural blueprints and terminology. In
the past five years, I have become inti-
mately involved with architects in developing space requirements and working drawings for a 4½ million dollar comprehensive community mental health center, for
inpatient and day hospital units in two
community hospitals, and for a geriatric
village on the grounds of a facility for
elderly persons. In order for an architect to formulate effective architectural
plans for a mental health program he needs
the assistance of a mental health professional who can not only spell out a viable program in terms the architect can
comprehend but who also understands the
language and drawings of architects and
the construction industry.

h) Coordinator

A prime mental health administrator
role is that of coordinator. This involves
coordination in program planning and direction between clinic directors and local
boards of mental health associations, between the area professional staff and area
citizen boards, between professionals in
different facilities operating in the same
geographic area, and between regional and
area-wide facilities. It is essential, as
comprehensive community mental health programs develop and expand, that the numerous groups who are involved learn to co-
operate and collaborate with each other.
At times friction develops and the regional mental health administrator is called
in to mediate the conflict; at other times
the mental health administrator is asked

to serve as an advocate for local clinics
or citizen boards who are seeking community recognition and support for their
programs. On still other occasions his
help as a resource person is requested.
To be effective in this role the mental
health administrator must be perceived
as knowledgeable and cooperative and, at
the same time, objective and fair minded
in mediating differences which may arise
between groups.

i) Expeditor

        Related to the coordinator function
is the expeditor role. It is not merely
sufficient to orchestrate the harmonious
operation of a community-wide network of
mental health and retardation services,
it is also essential to facilitate the
forward progress of planning and implementation of needed new or modified programs. If a program or if planning gets
bogged down it is the task of the administrator to discover the nature of the resistance, to unfreeze the status quo, and
to get things moving again.

j) Conceptualizer

        In representing diverse professional
and citizen groups in the community the
mental health administrator has to help
not only in the planning, implementation,
and facilitation of programs, but also in
the conceptualization of the mental health
goals of the area. He must deal with such
questions as: What are the mental health
goals and objectives of the area? How
does one establish priorities? How does
one institute change? How does one deal

with resistance to change? How does one
assess the impact of existing programs?
How does one determine the appropriateness of different models in a mental
health service delivery system? How does
one implement ideas? This role is suited
to a psychologist who has been trained in
conceptual analysis, in an understanding
of human development and behavior, in a
grasp of motivational determinants, and
in experiences in dyadic relationships.
The more the administrator possesses these
qualities the better he will be able to
perform this difficult aspect of his job.

k) Fund Raising

      I have appeared on numerous occasions
before mayors, selectmen, adlermen, town
councils, boards of health, and school
committees at the behest of local mental
health and mental retardation associations
and area citizen boards to aid in their
quest of obtaining local funds to support
their programs. Especially in these days
of "tight" public money, it is vital that
city and town officials understand the
importance and place of preventive and
rehabilitative mental health programs in
their overall community priorities of
needs. An effective mental health administrator must possess the knowledge and
expertise to assist in that process.

l) Personnel Recruiter

      An important administrative function
is the search for and recruitment of qualified professionals to fill key positions
in clinics and state hospitals. When I
go to professional conventions I invari-

ably spend at least a day at the placement
section talking to job applicants and assessing their qualifications. Every day
I receive numerous resumes from persons
seeking jobs. My office staff screens
them, catalogues them, discusses them with
me, and makes appropriate applicants' resumes available to those facilities in the
region which have vacant positions.

The administrator also serves on
search committees which are established
to select professionals for key positions,
such as a director of a mental health center or a superintendent of a state hospital or school. The selection and appointment of highly qualified persons to
operate the facilities over which he has
jurisdiction is important to the administrator in helping him achieve his goals.

m) Budget Analyst

As administrator of a regional office
I am accountable for the expenditure of
over 30 million dollars for the operation
of state hospitals, state schools, mental
health clinics, nursery schools for ex-
ceptional children, and a variety of other
programs. Six separate budgets are submitted each year to the regional office
for review, for critical suggestions, and
for approval (or disapproval). While the
mental health administrator is not expected to be a fiscal expert (he has a business manager to handle the technical de-
tails of budget expenditures) it is in-
cumbent upon him to understand thoroughly
all aspects of the budget process including budget preparation, budget appropria-
tions, transfers from one account to an-

other, deficiency and supplementary budget requests, etc. The budget is the lu-
bricant which enables programs to flourish
(or founder), to expand (or decay), to innovate (or to remain stagnant). With the
present money crisis and limited budgets,
crucial decisions have to be made regarding reductions in programs, services, and
overhead costs. For example, in my region
we now require about 35 million dollars
to maintain our current level of operations. However, the Governor recommended
(and the legislature approved) only 30
million dollars in the 1974 fiscal year
budget. Thus, five million dollars has
to be pared in some manner in order to
keep within the appropriation limits.
Crucial questions have to be resolved regarding which programs to cut back, which
services to reduce, which overhead functions to trim, and how economies can be
effected with the least devastating impact on existing programs and services.
Difficult decisions have to be made--the
better the administrator understands the
intricacies of the budget process, the
better he will be able to make these decisions.

n) Planned Change Agent

     The mental health administrator is
frequently asked to participate in task
forces or boards of organizations which
are concerned with changing health and/or
mental health systems. For example, at
present I am on a task force, organized
jointly by the United Community Services
of Boston and the Department of Mental
Health, which is charged with planning
the future role of the state mental hos-

pital in the Commonwealth as the deinstitutionalization of patients from the hospital to community-based facilities begins
to accelerate. I was formerly on the
Board of the Health Planning Council of
Greater Boston which has a mandate to plan
for health delivery systems in the Metropolitan Boston area. Recently, I was asked to be on the board of a PSRO (Professional Standards Review Organization)
which will attempt to evaluate the professional performance of medical practitioners. Participation in these groups
ensures at least some input into the planned change process and is an important
function of the mental health administrator's role.

o)   Inspector and Standard Setter

        In conjunction with the state in-
spector of hospital facilities, I make
periodic visits to the state and private
psychiatric hospitals in my region to determine whether they are abiding by the
regulations of the Department regarding
the care, treatment, and civil rights of
patients and whether they meet the standards set forth by national accrediting
agencies. In those instances where regulations are not followed or standards are
not met, these institutions are required
to submit a plan for compliance. The assistance of the regional administrator
and his office is made available to help
institutions upgrade standards and comply
with state regulations. The regional administrator has the authority to recommend
the suspension or withholding of a license
to a private psychiatric facility until
such time as it meets the appropriate

standards.

p) Primary Prevention Facilitator

Another role of the regional administrator is that of facilitator of primary
prevention approaches to mental health.
The natural tendency of professionals and
the public, especially when money is in
short supply, is to emphasize those programs which offer treatment and rehabilitation to mentally ill, emotionally disturbed, and mentally retarded persons,
and to minimize those programs that attempt to assess causes for diseases, disorders, and maladjustment processes or
that attempt to anticipate those emotional problems which are likely to occur in
populations at risk. Persons who are currently emotionally or mentally incapaci-
tated **are** the most visible and it is natural to want to alleviate their distress.
We could double or triple the amount we
now spend and still not meet all the needs
of these people. Persons with incipient
emotional or mental problems are somewhat
less visible and there is the tendency to
let them muddle through as best they can.
I'm referring to persons who present some
problems in school, some difficulties in
holding a job, some depression in middle
age, some adjustment problems at retirement. While we recognize that these persons are not enjoying the full fruits of
a satisfying life, they somehow manage to
avoid institutionalization or professional
psychiatric help. The persons who are in
need of some mental health program but who
are least visible to the planners are
those individuals who are going through
critical developmental stages in their

life as well as those persons whose economic, social, or cultural environment
renders them more susceptible to break-
down under the stresses and strains of
daily living than their neighbors who are
not confronted by such intense environmental pressures. I'm referring to persons who come from broken homes or de-
prived households; those faced daily with
poverty or low standards of living; those
encountering emotional stresses due to alcohol, drugs, bereavement, divorce, or
death of loved ones; those facing such
developmental crises as beginning school,
entering adolescence, getting married,
having children, going through the meno-
pause, having children leave to go to college or to marry, or facing the declining
years of life. Primary intervention ad-
dresses itself to the anticipation of emotional problems and tries to ward them off
or at least to minimize their impact on
the individual's state of emotional health
in the future. The importance of primary
prevention is becoming increasingly recognized as an integral part of comprehensive
mental health planning. The task before
us is to develop viable primary prevention
programs. The mental health administrator
can play an important role in educating
his colleagues to the merits of primary
prevention efforts and in facilitating the
development of such programs through his
influence over budgetary priorities.

An example of a primary prevention
effort is the behavioral science teaching
program which was initiated about eight
years ago as a collaborative venture between the South Shore Mental Health Clinic
and the Quincy, Massachusetts, schools. A

series of behavioral science curricula
was developed for elementary school children from kindergarten to sixth grade.
Three areas were covered: 1) explanation
of the learning process, 2) principles of
physical growth and development, and 3)
understanding of moods and emotions. The
presentations were given in an informal
manner and free group discussion was encouraged. Topics such as intelligence and
aptitude, individual differences in rates
of learning, and psychological factors af-
fecting the learning process were included
in the first area. Discussions of differences in weight and height, activity rates,
and genetic characteristics were pertinent
to the second area. Free discussions and
stories relating to feelings, moods, and
emotions of anger, sibling rivalry, shy-
ness, etc. were part of the third area.
Many children discussed the behavioral
science sessions with their parents, some
of whom expressed an interest in learning
more about this subject matter themselves.
As a result, a parents' group was formed.

It is difficult to measure the long-
term impact of this primary prevention
experiment but the program still continues (in modified form) to this day. Informal assessment measures appeared to
demonstrate favorable results on such variables as better understanding of one's
feelings, better relationships with peers
and family members, and better control
over aggressive and socially unacceptable
behavior.

q) Evaluator

Last, but far from least, is the role

of the mental health administrator as an evaluator of mental health and retardation programs. This is an area which has been sorely neglected in the state mental health system and which receives only a pittance out of a total budget of 175 million dollars that the state allots to the Department of Mental Health. As costs increase and money becomes scarcer, increasing attention is being paid to evaluation of existing mental health programs. In my region, I have required that all requests for the funding of new programs include an evaluation component with a detailed explanation of how the evaluation will be built in and implemented during the life of the program. In order to facilitate this process, I plan to make available the resources of a consultant who is skilled in program evaluation. Also, some external evaluation process will be instituted to supplement the program's internal evaluation procedure.

Evaluation is an essential aspect of program development. It is not enough merely to conceptualize programs, to plan programs, or to implement programs; it is also necessary to assess the efficacy of those programs. We can no longer afford to operate programs indefinitely; we must be prepared to eliminate or reduce those services which are less effective and to develop or expand others which show promise.

THE FUTURE OF MENTAL HEALTH ADMINISTRATION

Heraclitus, the Greek philosopher, once remarked that the only thing that is

permanent is change. In this context it
is interesting to speculate on two major
changing directions the mental health administrator role is likely to take during
the next five years or so (Rosenblum,
1972).

First, it appears probable that his
primary role will be that of contracting
with private, nonprofit groups to implement programs which have been developed
by mental health professionals in con-
junction with local citizen groups. The
mental health administrator will likely
continue to assist in the process of program conceptualization, program planning,
program development, program implementation, standard setting, and program evaluation while nongovernmental agencies will
be selected to operate the programs and
to be accountable annually to the mental
health administrator for their quality
and effectiveness.

The other future role for the mental
health administrator is his participation
in a larger human services delivery system as an administrator for both public
health and mental health programs. This
new administrator role will require close
collaboration with other human services
departments such as welfare, rehabilitation, corrections, elderly affairs, and
youth services to achieve a network of
services which will integrate the total
needs of an individual, from economic to
physical needs to psychological and social needs. There will be a gradual shift
from a medical model of providing services
which calls for M.D.'s, Ph.D.'s, M.S.W.'s,
and RN's to a broad psychosociological

model which utilizes paraprofessionals and nonprofessionals, as well as professionally-trained persons, in administering and providing for a broad range of human needs in a multiservice setting. Within this context I see an exciting and promising future for community psychologists as human services coordinators and facilitators as well as community and mental health administrators.

EPILOGUE

I should like to address myself briefly to a dilemma which often besets a new mental health administrator who comes from a clinical background. Hirschowitz (1971) has labeled this as the "clinician-executive" dilemma in which a clinical stance which serves the person well in a medical or psychological setting becomes a crippling bind for planning and executive functions. The clinician who practices an analytic or nondirective approach to clinical situations may find himself at a loss when placed in an administrative role which requires swift political responses, direct action, and negotiation with community agencies. The administrator, unlike the clinician, says Hirschowitz, is much more than a reactor; he is an interactor, a proactor, and a transactor. To a degree he has to unlearn aspects of the posture and style he may have acquired as a clinician. Whittington (1969) makes the following cogent comments about the liabilities of a clininal stance in executing a mental health administrator's function:

As social planners, our impatience
and rudeness do not endear us to
others in community action groups.
Our role as king whose legitimacy is
challenged makes us vulnerable to
self-doubt, anxiety, and paranoia
/p. 458/.

The clinican-administrator dilemma
is best resolved, according to Hirschowitz (1971),

when the administrator learns to adopt
an appropriate, flexible role repertoire which avoids role clinging. If
he knows his community, if he knows
how, where, and when to move, how to
negotiate and trade in the corridors
of power, he will find growth-enab-
ling solutions to his leadership dilemmas /p. 115/.

REFERENCES

Hirschowitz, R. G. Dilemmas of leadership in community mental health. Psychiatric Quarterly, 1971, 45, 102-116.

Rosenblum, G. Mental health retools for
the 70's. Massachusetts Journal of Mental Health, 1972, 2, 5-16.

Whittington, H. G. Institutional lodg-
ment of the community mental health center. American Journal of Public Health,
1969, 59, 458-461.

4. THE EDUCATING OF A
COMMUNITY PSYCHOLOGIST

Edison J. Trickett

My conception of the general mandate
for this series is that I am to summarize
my own professional development in the
area we call community psychology and
point out current problems and future prospects of this area as I perceive them.
Since I see the current problems as multiple and the future prospects as uncer-
tain, there is much to talk about. I
welcome this opportunity to do so in the
context of other talks which may yield
a perspective more rosy than mine.

First a word about my own perspec-
tives--where I'm coming from personally
as well as institutionally. Like many
who identify themselves as community psychologists, my own graduate training was
that of a clinician, mirroring the assumptions of the Boulder conference of
the late 1940's. Like my fellow students at Ohio State, I was to be a scien-
tist/professional who could teach, conduct research, and act--a kind of triple-
threat clinician's clinician. I remember

much of my training, its content and process, not as much fondly as vividly. On the fond side was George Kelly, who taught philosophy of science, in my mind a <u>sine qua non</u> for any breed of psychologist. Psychopathology, diagnostic testing, psychotherapy--individual and group--were the core intellectual experiences, liberally spiced with survey-ish courses in child development and social psychology. Of course, homage was paid to both methodology and statistics in that both were "required." However, the methodology and statistics had their own built-in bigotry about the requirements of "tight" research. Thus, for example, field methods were never mentioned by our profoundly intelligent and witty professor Reed Lawson, and multivariate statistics were generally seen as "unnecessary" for us clinicians.

I labor over the content of environmental press operative in my own training program to underscore an important and recurrent problem for a field which has yet to develop conceptually sound and experientially integrated training programs; namely, that postgraduate work is not so much a clear extension of one's graduate training as a kind of retraining for ways of thinking <u>and</u> ways of behaving not internalized from the course content nor socialized by the <u>in vivo</u> experiences of clinical training.

The research enterprise at Ohio State was similarly solid though somewhat confining. The press was on laboratory studies, the manipulation of variables, and the general intensive study of the college sophomore. Recent content analyses of ar-

ticles appearing in the Journal of Personality and Social Psychology suggest
little change in this convenient, experimentally-based means of accruing knowledge (Highbee & Wells, 1972). Again, I
mention this thrust not to play down an
approach which has yielded valuable insights and public, verifiable, reproducible findings, but to round out where I
came from for the purpose of later contrast in terms of some directions in which
community psychology, in my judgment,
needs to focus its intellectual energies.

One ripple in the otherwise smooth
flow of assumptions surrounding clinical
training was Jim Kelly. Jim had received
clinical training, but had added a Masters in Public Health from Harvard and
experience at the National Institute of
Mental Health. His lexicon focused more
on resources than psychological defenses,
more on interdependence than nosological
schemes, more on situational determinants
and person-setting interactions than personality traits, and more on prevention
or positive socialization goals than remediation or treatment of casualties.
This general thrust, more specifically
embodied in what Jim called the "ecological analogy," was not in the zeitgeist of
Ohio State in the mid-1960's, however, and
Jim moved to Michigan. I finished my doctorate at Ohio State but under his supervision. Yet in this process my own career
had taken a turn toward clarification
which gave it a more syntonic quality than
had existed in the more clinical aspects
of my training. This was true both for
research and practice. With respect to
the former, I decided to pursue the study

of people in contexts and the study of
contexts themselves; with respect to "doing something about it," my decision was
to focus on the process and content of
consultation and other intervention strategies as they related to socialization
environments and their members.

Having embarked on a new set of assumptions about behavior, on a new level
of analysis--the assessment of settings
and person-setting interactions--and on
thoughts on change not rooted in psychotherapeutic strategies of intervention, I
felt ill-equipped to commit myself to ei-
ter of two prime options: joining an academic faculty in psychology or working for
a community mental health center. Fortunately, I found the ideal alternative
in a two-year postdoctoral research fel-
lowship at Stanford Medical Center working with Rudolf Moos. Rudy had been vig-
orously pursuing research in two areas of
direct interest to me: the source of behavioral variance accounted for by person,
setting, and person-setting interaction;
and the assessment of environments. Here
was the chance to sharpen my thinking in
areas of importance without getting en-
meshed in administrative activities or
other commitments to program-building
which take such an extraordinary toll of
time and energy, and a chance to become
involved in research on problem areas
which I felt--and still feel--are pivotal
to the development of an adequate knowledge base for a psychology of the community. I decided to forestall active efforts at creating change in favor of working on conceptions and simply acquiring
knowledge. I was frankly worried that the

personal satisfaction in "being where the
action is" and of doing work that God
knows needed doing would have taken too
great an unintended toll on my ability to
work out conceptual frameworks and perspectives. In short, my observing ego
might have been permanently arrested.

Be that as it may, I began at Stanford the lines of research which have oc-
cupied me to the present day. Let me
describe them at some length and link
them up to some general set of ideas surrounding my conception of community psychology.

PERSON-ENVIRONMENT INTERACTIONS

The first area of work involved a
foray into person-environment interactions. It was initially stimulated by
the work of Harold Raush in a series of
papers describing situational influences
on two groups of boys: one "emotionally
disturbed" and one "normal" (Raush, Dittman, & Taylor, 1959a, 1959b). Analysis
of the behavior of both groups indicated
significant setting effects and person x
setting interactions. Later work by Hunt
and Endler confirmed these kinds of effects for the traits of anxiety and hostility (e.g., Endler & Hunt, 1968). This
general line of inquiry was congruent with
my stance toward community psychology in
several ways. First, my assumption was
that "people in context," people in the
natural settings where they live and work,
were an appropriate focus for community
psychology. This, then, raised a number
of issues about the influence of settings

on behavior and on person by setting interaction as both a research domain and
a conceptual stance. If, for example, interaction effects were shown to be minimal, then the conceptual stance clearly
suffers.

There was a second compelling reason
why this area was of initial interest;
namely, that at this time, as now, I see
one paramount issue in community psychology as involving the conceptualization
and assessment of communities or subunits
of communities which we may call, after
Sarason (1972), "settings." But settings,
of course, are only important if, indeed,
they exercise a demonstrable effect across
all participants and/or if these are significant interactions which account for
not only statistically significant but
psychologically meaningful amounts of behavioral variance. If, as I believe, the
level of analysis of behavior most germane
to community psychology was not the individual level on which much clinical training was based, but instead dealt with the
"main effect" of institutions on people
or defined behavior as an interactive consequence of people with personal characteristics X and Y and settings having Z
demand characteristics, then this line of
inquiry seemed essential.

At this point, I made the choice to
concentrate my research efforts in and on
a particular institution, the public
school. While theorizing about such areas
as person-setting interaction is appropriately seen as a general problem in the
understanding of behavior (i.e., interaction effects don't occur only at school)

I decided to use the school as my particular locus of concern. This choice was
conceptually consistent with my view of
community psychology as concerned less
with remediation and more with prevention,
or indeed the enhancement of positive socialization goals. The general reason-
ing was that public schools are the only
public institutions which: (1) require
that children or youth attend; (2) are
explicitly concerned with normative questions regarding the education and psychosocial development of children and youth;
and (3) are both encouraged and mandated
to provide necessary remediation. Being
concerned with promoting development, public schools are somewhat different than
mental hospitals, correctional facilities,
psychiatric clinics, or storefronts.
These are, on the institutional level,
agencies of what Caplan calls tertiary
or perhaps secondary prevention. For better or worse, then, public schools capture
and socialize youth: they can be con-
ceived of as communities struggling to
perform such community tasks as developing indigenous resources and adapting to
neighboring communities. They can, and
have, served many truly community functions, both educational and political.

The choice to locate my research efforts in a particular kind of setting had
pragmatic overtones as well; namely, that
I wanted to begin to generate an experiential data base for later work in psychological consultation. I wanted to see
how schools as institutions functioned,
how they might be similar to or different than mental hospitals, and what kinds
of factors internal to schools might con-

strain the effectiveness of varied interventions.

This dual motivation resulted in my
adopting a research stance that implies
a real tension and one which, on occasion,
forces one to trade off some intellectual
curiosity about a more general body of
knowledge in favor of learning about a
particular institutional expression of a
more general phenomenon. Said another
way, this is a tension between pursuing
a phenomenon (e.g., dissonance theory)
which presumably cuts across content
areas, subjects and situations, and pursuing the understanding of that phenomenon in a particular setting (e.g., the
school). This is not necessarily a basic-
applied distinction, but rather more of
a concern with what has been called the
"ecological validity" of research findings concerning presumably general phenomena. My decision, for the time being,
was to remain setting-determined in my
research, working in the schools and investigating aspects of the person-environment relationship in that context.

Let me give one example of a study
constructed to investigate both a general
phenomenon and to learn about setting-
specific implications at the same time.
In a nonschool-related research effort,
Rudy Moos and I were interested in the
relationship of self-other perceived similarity and satisfaction with the environment (Trickett & Moos, 1972). The metho-
dology--stimulated by the work of Lawrence
Pervin--was to ask inmates in a correctional institution to rate themselves,
their ideal selves, and various reference

groups (e.g., guards, other inmates) on
a semantic differential. We computed difference scores based on the discrepancy
between self-rating and each reference
group rating, correlating this discrepancy with their responses on several items
asking them how satisfied they were with
different groups in their immediate environment. The findings strongly confirmed that perceived similarity to a
particular reference group is most strongly related to satisfaction with that reference group, but not to general satisfaction or satisfaction with another reference group.

What if we do a similar study using
the school and its relevant reference
groups of teachers, close friends, other
kids at school, etc.--as a demonstration
of the generalizability of this phenomenon. We can not only gather such data
across a new set of conditions and across
another sample, we can also include areas
of inquiry which can lend insight into the
specifics of schools (see Carew, 1973, for
a complete report).

As a couple of examples of this, let
us take two questions included in the
school study which yielded specific information beyond the domain of the general relationship of perceived self-environment similarity to satisfaction. One
question involves a pivotal function--as
I see it--of schools. Stated simply, it
is whether or not schools are perceived
by students as helping them fulfill personal goals. In terms of the research,
the question was thus: is there a relationship between perceived similarity to

various reference groups and the likeli-
hood that school is seen as facilitative
in this regard? We found the answer to
be _yes_, but with some cogent developmental differences between freshmen and seniors. For freshmen, only perceived similarity to teachers related to experiencing school as helpful in fulfilling personal goals. Teachers were also important for seniors, but in addition, similarity to peers also related to whether
or not they see school as goal fulfilling.
Thus, across developmental levels, identification of teachers as similar to oneself is an important ingredient in one's
assessment of schools along this dimension.

A second question involved what we
called "spillover," although this term
implies a causal relationship which we
could not directly test in our correla-
tional data. It dealt with the issue--
an issue raised in the earlier correctional study--of whether or not similarity to any specific reference groups was
related to a more general satisfaction
with the environment as a whole. We found
no consistent relationship in the correctional institution study, but we did when
applying the same question across two age
levels in schools. In short, general satisfaction with the school was consistent-
ly related to perceived similarity to
teachers, but not to peers, even among
seniors. Our own speculation about these
two findings is that teachers seem to
emerge as quite influential figures, far
more so than peers, in relating to the
quality of student satisfactions with
school.

Returning to the original question of why investigate a particular phenomenon of interest in one setting rather than another, I hope that the above data supplies at least a partial rationale; namely, that one can learn something more theoretically general as well as its setting-specific ramifications if attention is thusly focused. Because my interests were both conceptual and pragmatic, this stance seemed particularly valid.

I also attempted another methodology to pursue the person-setting interaction more directly. The prior studies seemed to affirm the importance of conceptualizing behavior in terms of a "fit" between self-perception and perception of the environment, but did not address directly the key question of how much variance is accounted for by person, by setting, and by person-setting interaction. Data was indeed available from Raush's earlier work and from the questionnaire studies by Endler and Hunt on the traits of anxiety and hostility. Endler and Hunt provided the statistical rationale, but used predominantly hypothetical situations. Raush provided information on "live behavior," but did not analyze the data in ways which specified amount of variance accounted for by person, setting, and interaction. The ideal test would have included behavioral observations coded in terms of response categories which could be analyzed via the Endler-Hunt three-way analysis of variance. As is often the case, only lack of money prevented us from doing this. We regressed to the questionnaire and, staying in the schools, found 12 students who shared four classes. We asked them to rate their reactions in these four classes along several dimensions, including: "paying attention," "participation," "anxiety," and "satisfaction." Each response dimension was characterized by several items. We then analyzed the data using a three-way analysis of variance for each response dimension, allowing us to specify for each dimension the amount of variance accounted for by each of the three main effects (students, classes, and response dimensions) and their interactions. We then calculated the relative percentages of total variance accounted for by each source for each response dimension. The results provided no surprises as they essentially supported earlier work, but now within the context of the school (Trickett & Moos, 1970). The most interesting result was that for every response dimension, the interaction of Person x Setting accounted for the largest proportion of variance, ranging from 30 percent to 50 percent. Setting or situational differences also accounted for statistically significant amounts of variance. For example, Math class satisfies students significantly less than does English class.

Taken seriously, such questionnaire data have led to interesting action implications in our consultation work in schools (see O'Neill & Trickett, 1973), and I can without fear of contradiction say that they have been experientially validated--students who are referred for psychological help inevitably find some adaptive niche as they pass through the school day. Interaction effects are great, although we are just beginning to look at

what some of the contributors to these
effects are.

In any case, these small, though useful, studies helped give me an orientation
toward person-environment interdependence
which at least raised useful questions in
assessing in vivo behavior and which have
led in subsequent years to implications
for how consultants conceive of problems
and behave in their problem-solving roles.

AN ECOLOGICAL PERSPECTIVE AND
THE ASSESSMENT OF ENVIRONMENTS

From this general set of questions
about "where" behavior comes from (e.g.,
is its determination personological, situational, or interactional), my research
and thinking turned toward a related and,
for me, more compelling set of questions.
My training had provided me with a reasonably solid conception about the nature of
people and the assessment, in a variety
of ways, of their personalities and behavior. But the level of analysis was
shifting to people in context or the contexts themselves. Community psychology,
by semantic implication, signifies a community of one sort or another as some kind
of entity with its own properties worthy
of study in its own right. Thus, the
quest turned toward varied ways of assessing settings, again a pursuit far from
my clinical heritage. I have subsequently spent considerable time looking at two
general notions of environmental assessment, one heavily empirical and one--the
ecological analogy--tremendously useful
on a heuristic level, though in need of

concretization. Let me briefly outline
these two different approaches. First,
the work on perceived environment.

Perceived Environment and the Classroom Environment Scale

My original interest in looking at
environment through the eyes of participants in that environment stemmed from
the work of Henry Murray and his notion
of beta press (Murray, 1939) as that aspect of the environment agreed on or shared
by people--the "consensual" environment.
More specifically, the empirical strivings
of Stern and Pace to assess college atmos-
pheres (Stern, 1970) gave a general orientation to this area. All this was rein-
forced, however, by the line of inquiry
Rudy Moos was, and still is, taking.
Briefly, Rudy was about the business of
developing measures of the perceived environment of various human service settings, first the psychiatric ward and then
with halfway houses, correctional institution living units, and others. To re-
capitulate, I was very interested in this
area, but particularly as it may be applied to educational settings. I decided
to use the high school classroom as a setting, and we set out to create the Classroom Environment Scale (Trickett & Moos,
1973; Moos & Trickett, 1973) in the following way. First, true to my academic
heritage, a literature review was undertaken to investigate different ways of
looking at classrooms. Second, we review-
ed popular literature such as Up the Down
Staircase (Kaufman, 1965) to see if we
could learn anything. Finally, we sat in
on classes in surrounding public schools

and interviewed teachers and students in-
tensively on the nature of their classroom experiences. We ended up with numerous piles of dimensions, descriptive
phrases, and summarized research reports.
Yet our multiple methods for gathering
this information paid off in some interesting ways. For example, there was some
overlap, but certainly no exact corres-
pondence, between the aspects of the classroom defined by researchers as salient and
those defined as salient by students.

We ended up viewing the classroom as
a social system with four general aspects:
(1) the authority function inherent in the
teacher role and manifested not only in
the strictness and clarity of rules; but
in the degree of order and organization
present in the classroom; (2) the friendship function of the teacher in dealings
with students in terms of personal support
of students and in general student involvement in the class; (3) the peer-peer relationships, particularly how well students
got along with each other and cooperated
around class activities or projects; and
(4) the function-specific variables of the
classroom, those relating to the academic
goals of the classroom. In our work these
turned out to be Competition for grades
and honors among students, and Task Ori-
entation--how much the class stuck to the
learning task at hand and did not get distracted. We all probably remember teachers from our own school days who, when the
weather was beautiful or the topic particularly boring, could be distracted from
the lesson or even be convinced to call
off class. It is this kind of dimension
that Task Orientation was after.

Having arrived at this general conception, we started our empirical phase by
generating literally hundreds of items
describing about 15 dimensions of the high
school classroom. For example, "Almost
all class time is spent on the lesson for
the day" was one item reflecting the more
general concept of Task Orientation.
Wherever possible we tried to use verba-
tim statements from teachers and students.
The results of this "statement-writing"
made it clear that some selectivity was
called for: no one with any conscience
would ask high school students to respond
to 500 or more items about the same classroom. We ended up by selecting 242 items
--still, perhaps, a morally questionable
amount--which by a priori conceptual relevance, fit into one of 13 general dimensions. These items, which were set in
a true-false format, could be completed
in a regular classroom period, as we discovered by giving it in 26 high school
classes. Once these initial data were
collected, one-way analyses of variance
were done on each item across the 26 classrooms. If an item did not differentiate,
or distinguish, among the 26 classrooms,
it was discarded. Even after this analysis was completed and the appropriate
items dropped, we had a large number of
items on all but one of the 13 dimensions.
Using the remaining data, we intercorre-
lated the subscales; the primary finding
emerging from this was that the mind can
make logical conceptual distinctions which,
while remaining distinct in the head of
conceptualizer, are nevertheless so highly
correlated in nature as to be interchange-
able. A good example is the subscale entitled Order and Organization. Original-

ly, the conception was that <u>Order</u> would
refer essentially to level of classroom
uproar or noise level and that <u>Organiza-
tion</u> would refer to how organized the
teacher was in preparing for class, or-
ganizing lessons, etc.   Conceptually these
two dimensions were distinct, but in the
real world of classrooms, they are highly
related. Thus, they were collapsed into
one dimension on the final scale.

As a result of our first effort we
were left with a number of dimensions that
looked empirically solid, but we still had
not "captured" some of the concepts we
felt were important. Thus we gave it another try, generating additional items and
reworking some of the concepts in light
of the first administration. We then presented another version of the scale (Form
C) with a reduced number of items, mostly
old but some new, to another sample of
over 20 classrooms. This time we got it.
Again, the one-way analysis of variance
was conducted on each item. Over 95 percent of the items significantly differentiated between the classrooms. On the
basis of subscale intercorrelations we
decided on nine dimensions of the classroom: <u>Student Involvement</u> in the classroom; <u>Innovation</u> in approaches to teaching; <u>Teacher Support</u> of students on a personal level; Student-Student <u>Affiliation</u>;
<u>Teacher Control</u>, a less negatively charged
way of describing <u>Rule Strictness</u>, which
meant essentially what it said; <u>Rule Cla-
rity</u>, which as a distinct dimension correlated slightly over .3 with Teacher Control; and <u>Task Orientation</u> and Student-
<u>Student Competition</u>, which represented the
goal orientation variables of the class-

room. Final selection of items for each
of the nine dimensions were based on several criteria, including moderate to high
item-subscale correlation, breadth of content within a specified dimension, and
the obvious stipulation that every item
correlate more highly with its own subscale than with any other subscale. We
ended up with 10 items per dimension,
usually half keyed true and half keyed
false, with an average dimension inter-
correlation of about .25, ranging from
essentially no correlation to a high of
.51 between any two dimensions.

We have collected over 300 classrooms
worth of data (about 6000 students) by
now for a normative sample worthy of the
name. In this process we are beginning
to learn a fair amount about classrooms.
We know, for example, that math and science classes are far more Task-Oriented
and have less Teacher Support than do English classes. We don't know, however,
whether the difference is related more to
the class content or the personality of
teachers who opt for math/science or English (Moos & Trickett, 1973). We know
that a systematic relationship exists between perceived classroom environment and
student satisfaction with the classroom
(Trickett & Moos, 1973).

Further, we believe that a predict-
ble relationship exists between the goals
one has for an environment and the kind
of classroom atmosphere one might attempt
to create. For example, if one is interested in a generally satisfied class, the
environmental correlates appear to include
Teacher Support, Student Involvement, and

Rule Clarity. If one values learning a
great deal of content, however, additional environmental dimensions--most vividly, Competition--seem to become involved.
Thus, while speculative, it appears that
a meaningful relationship exists between
the goals of a setting and the psychosocial atmosphere, with the implication that
as one changes, the other changes.

Perceived Environment and Change

In addition to personal correlates
of perceived environment, we are working
with two different models of change using
the concept of perceived environment and
related measures, a stance consistent with
the assertion that community psychology
analyzes not the individual so much as the
setting or person-setting interaction. In
our current jargon, these two approaches
are labelled "Discrepancy Model" and "Criterion Model." The Discrepancy Model is
essentially based on the discrepancy between "real" perceived environment and
consensual "ideal" environment. At Stanford, we attempted this with moderate success and, as often occurs in in vivo
change-oriented research, with less than
optimal methodological rigor, on a psychiatric ward (Pierce, Trickett, & Moos,
1971). Patients and staff filled out
"real" and "ideal" measures of the perceived environment and used feedback from
the analyzed data to focus discussion
about change on the ward and to pinpoint
specific aspects of the environment where
the "real" and the "ideal" diverged. This
basically descriptive information was seen
as helpful in articulating a frame of reference within which people could "locate"

their gripes and joys about the place.
Indeed, it brought out some people who
had previously been identified as silent
members of the culture. Various change
strategies were discussed, and several
action plans emerged. Several months later we again assessed the perceived environment to see if the gap between the
real and the ideal had narrowed, which it
had. An interesting study shortly after,
by the way, found that engaging in the
change program had changed peoples' conception of the "ideal" environment as well
as their perception of the real (Cooper,
1973).

The second approach, the "Criterion
Model," is from the work of Ben Schneider,
currently at the University of Maryland.
This model involves the prior specifica-
tion of single or multiple criteria which
one is concerned about and constructing
a measure of the perceived environment to
see what aspects of the environment relate most strongly to the criteria. Essentially three steps are postulated within this information-processing framework.
First come observations of rather specific events in the environment; second,
perceptual "conclusions" are arrived at
based on those events; third, decisions
about action--in Schneider's work, the
decision of whether or not to switch banks
--result from these perceptual conclusions.
Locating these perceptual antecedents of
specified criteria can serve to define
changes appropriate to the situation.
Summarizing implications for change,
Schneider (1972, p. 19) states:

The framework enables the researcher
to predict perceiver behavior, and
also permits identification of the
specific elements of the situation
on which climate perceptions are based.
By examining these elements, changes
which may result in altered climate
perceptions can be specified.

Perceptual changes are seen as means to
changing consequent behaviors.

While we have not as yet directly
utilized the Classroom Environment Scale
in attempting either of these possible
change strategies, the most important
point is the applicability of measures of
perceived environment to an important problem of community psychology: namely, the
assessment of settings and the utility of
that assessment for setting change.

Ecological Analogy

The other approach for looking at
settings or communities was instigated by
Jim Kelly, helpfully augmented by Dave
Todd. It was an attempt to translate what
Jim called the "ecological analogy" to the
social organization of the high school, to
generate a way of thinking about communities using the high school as the relevant
subset (Trickett, Kelly, & Todd, 1972;
Trickett & Todd, 1972). Let me briefly
outline its meta-concepts and how it related to some of my work. I might add
that I have yet to find a set of concepts
which are as intellectually stimulating,
heuristically exciting and provocative,
and which focus the relevant questions in
such a stimulating way as does this ana-

logy.

Basically, as the name implies, the
ecological analogy involves a set of principles which research in field biology has
defined as valid for the study of naturally existing plant and animal communities.
The analogy asserts the appropriateness
of this perspective--a perspective refined
in the study of nonhuman communities--for
social organizations and man-made communities. Four additive principles are of
particular salience. These are: (1) Interdependence; (2) Adaptation; (3) Cycling
of Resources; and (4) Succession. Each
of these principles refers to unique properties or potentials of social environments, and adds increasing richness and
complexity to their assessment.

Interdependence. The principle of
interdependence asserts that the basic
elements of a system--such as roles, persons, policies, and settings--are dyna-
mically interrelated and that alterations
in one part of the social network will
induce change or reverberation in other
related parts. This principle directs
our attention to the context in which a
given behavior, role, or policy is embed-
ded as a basis for understanding or changing it. Specific solutions to problems
may have costly unanticipated consequences
elsewhere in the social environment if the
nature of this interdependence is not understood.

Within the context of the school, one
recent example comes quickly to mind. In
one school system in which we acted as
consultants, an assistant superintendent

of schools became disenchanted with the
guidance faculty at the high school. He
saw them as having very little to do.
(Needless to say his perception was not
shared by the guidance faculty.) In an
effort to "punish" them, he increased
their workload by making them accountable
for checking up on students who were tar-
dy or absent, a task previously undertaken by an assistant principal. One obvious problem became immediately clear to
guidance counselors and students alike:
the difficulty of maintaining the role of
confidante and friend to students while,
at the same time, being assigned a second
role as quasi-truant officer and watch-
dog. As a result, students increasingly
shunned the guidance counselor, instead
seeking comfort in the office of one of
the assistant principals who essentially
reversed roles with the guidance department, giving up part of his disciplinary
function to be a personal problem-solver.
Communication around these functions was
haphazard: on one occasion, a student's
guidance counselor discovered that guid-
ance-related topics were being discussed
in conferences between parents and the assistant principal, conferences of which
he had been unaware. Consequently, the
guidance counselors became increasingly
alienated from their new "truant-finding"
role and stopped checking up on absent
students. This essentially meant that
both the administration and the guidance
faculty did less surveillance on students
who failed to show up for school. Over
time, students learned that it was easier
to cut school with immunity, and "absen-
teeism" became defined as a problem. Such
an analysis--interminable I fear--could

continue, but suffice it to say that many
of the primary, though presumably unintended, consequences of this policy related to the nature of the role interdependence within the school.

An instance of a more explosive consequence of policy-making elsewhere was
that of a school board decision which, de
facto, discriminated against black students in a racially mixed high school
(Ochberg & Trickett, 1970). The decision
seemed to apply to all students, but the
issues--transportation on school buses to
and from school and elimination of hot
lunches--had different perceived effects
and real effects on black and white students. As an aside, one consequence of
this policy was to set in motion conditions which culminated in black-white
student confrontation and conflict.

It is this interdependence between
policies, roles, and individuals or informal groups which the interdependence
principle underlines.

Adaptation. The biological concept
of adaptation refers to the way in which
both individual organisms and species attempt to meet and condition the requirements of the environment for survival.
The translation of this principle has far-
reaching implications for the high school
setting, for it directs attention to the
institutional and interpersonal requirements for effective coping. It alerts
one to question what norms govern student
behavior; what roles and expected relationships constitute the "hidden curriculum"--to use Jackson's phrase--which

defines the socialization goals of the
school; and what behavioral roles are
available to students which lead to the
confirmation of identity, the attribution
of status, and accessibility to resources.

The concept of adaptation also directs attention to the reciprocal relationship between persons and settings by
embodying a view of personality as a set
of predispositions more or less responsive to differences in the behavioral requirements of settings. Consequently,
situational determinants of behavior
emerge as critical in the assessment process. It also suggests that because settings themselves have differing demand
characteristics, behavior which is effective in one setting may be maladaptive
in another. Thus, maintaining an effective and satisfying role requires a measure of "fit" between the personal qualities of individuals and the normative and
task requirements of the social system.

This principle clearly defines a perspective on social environments consistent
with assumptions underlying my earlier research on person-setting interaction and
that work relating to the assessment of
the perceived environment of the high
school classroom. In addition, as I mentioned previously, applied work as a psychological consultant has continuously
affirmed the relevance of this principle
not only for research but for practice.
In a minute I'll turn to its particular
applicability in terms of another area of
work--that relating to educational leadership during times of crisis.

Cycling of resources. In biology,
the cycling of resources refers to the
utilization and transformation of energy
through the life cycle of organisms in a
given habitat, how the nutrient material
circulated through this animal or plant
community serves as an indicator of the
life-sustaining processes of that habitat. In addition, the amount and distribution of resources relate to that
habitat's potential for perpetuation and
development. Related to the school, this
principle focuses on the quality and quan-
tity of available resources in the school
for defining and articulating problems,
meeting immediate needs, and developing
and expanding competencies. The manner
in which the school recruits, develops,
and utilizes such resources is thus a ba-
rometer of the extent and direction of
potential change in the school. This problem of creative development of indigenous talent is a critical concern for community psychologists--not simply the creating of training programs for paraprofessionals, college students, etc.,--but articulating the development of new resources
with the enhancing of the capacity of old
structures to perform new, often unreward-
ed functions within a specific context
(e.g., school or community).

The principle of cycling of resources
directs attention first at an assessment
of current functioning of various resources, formal and informal. In the area
of schools, for example, I believe such
basic descriptive information is incredi-
bly sparse. How much time, for example,
do $20,000-a-year principals spend doing
work which requires an eight-grade educa-

tion? How much do teachers differ in the
degree of out-of-class contact with students around personal problem-solving?
My experience with both these groups is
that the differences are considerable.
But personal experience is the common de-
nominator of us all in this area. We have
no data, we've developed no methodology;
indeed, we have just begun to develop an
articulatable concern with such resources,
especially as they apply to the broadly
defined area of the "helping" relationships existent in the school culture.
Surely a more sophisticated diagnosis and
evaluation of change would result from
finding out some of this descriptive information. I am reminded of Roger Barker's concern with our general lack of
baseline data in this respect, data about
what actually happens in peoples' lives,
what they actually do. If community psychology were to focus on some aspects of
this task--as I believe it should--the
principle of cycling of resources seems to
provide an extremely relevant set of questions.

   Succession. The biological principle of succession asserts that in the natural evolution of communities or habitats, the distribution of species changes
in response to the evolving demands of
the setting and its surrounding environment. In the present context, this concept is important in stressing the utility of a time perspective in the evolution of communities or schools as they
respond to and adapt to broader social,
technological, and demographic changes.
This time perspective includes two aspects: (a) an historical awareness of

the past events and personalities which
shape current norms, policies, and student characteristics; and (b) an anticipatory problem-solving perspective which
is future-oriented and planning-oriented.
In the assessment of environments, the
succession principle orients us toward
the means by which the social environment
assesses and copes with the impact of its
changing surroundings.

There are inherent problems in the
organizational structure of public schools
which make this principle a particularly
critical and interesting one in the area
of planning. As pointed out by Miles
(1967) and others such as Katz and Kahn
(1966), schools, unlike industry, generally have few institutional structures for
assessing the environment or getting feedback on how their "product" is doing.
They are not predicated on the need to
compete in order to survive. They are,
in Carlson's words, "domesticated" organizations. Part of this surely has to
do with having an assured clientele, and
part probably relates to the recurrent
difficulty of agreeing on and then measur-
ing educational "outputs."

Of course, the public school can
easily lapse into a collective mind set
which defends current efforts through ex-
ploiting this ambiguity about goals--a
kind of "How can we be failing if we can't
define what we're supposed to do?" perspective. But it also means that the institutional mechanisms for planning for
change--especially psychosocial change--
are absent, thus increasing the reliance
on individual school personnel to be ef-

fective visionaries. Nowhere is the lack
of planning engendered by this situation
more apparent than in public education's
efforts to cope with plans for integration. Familiar are the complaints that,
"I'm all for integration but I didn't know
it would be like this" or "The kids were
not ready for the school, the school was
not ready to deal with new behaviors or
attitudes toward authority," etc. Thus,
the Succession principle is peculiarly
important in the ways that it suggests
for conceptualizing aspects of public
schools.

Applicability of the Analogy

The elaboration of these four principles, particularly coupled with an extensive literature review, not only suggested exciting concepts, but asked questions relevant to community psychology
which were underrepresented in existing
literature on the assessment of settings
and theories of change. At this time, I
was experimenting with different methodologies appropriate to field research, with
one obvious approach being the case study. My clinical training had provided
some insights into the rules of the game
for understanding the cases of individuals: generally, these included a controlled environment for data gathering;
at least a minimal theoretical framework
--predominantly psychoanalytic ego psychology in my training; and a loose internal logic to rule hypotheses "in" or
"out."

In 1968, circumstances provided us
the opportunity to conduct a case study

evolving from the ecological analogy as
it applied to schools. California, sometimes with pride and sometimes dismay,
often serves as a warning to the rest of
the nation as to what social trends may
be expected, the Berkeley Free Speech
Movement being one example of a conspicu-
ous trend-setter. At this time, high
school unrest in the form of racial tensions and student power movements was an
unusually common occurrence in and around
Palo Alto. Frank Ochberg and I decided
that adopting a case study approach to
learning about high school disruption
would be pragmatic and intellectually stimulating at the same time. We soon realized, however, that to study schools qua
schools would require resources far beyond the most grandiose proposals of the
day. Partly out of our joint interest in
institutional leadership, and partly out
of serendipity, we chose to focus on the
high school principal who, above all,
should be in a position to view the school
as a small society and whose task functions should include constant barometric
readings of his kingdom. After collect-
ing narrative accounts of these situations,
mostly through interviews, we chanced upon
a reasonably rare opportunity to study a
school in some depth around the issue of
administrative coping with a student power
movement. The amount of information we
gathered made it pertinent to use the ecological analogy as a basis for directing
inquiry and discussing findings. Let me
give you briefly the context and flavor
of the inquiry derived from these ecological principles.

The previous year there had been a
rare principal who--by almost all reports
except those of student activists--dealt
competently and successfully with a student power movement spearheaded by several elected student leaders. Now "successfully" and "competently" mean quite
different things to different people. For
some people we talked to, "successfully"
meant "not letting the little bastards get
away with it," for some "competently" involved their perception of him as "on top
of things," as acting in accordance with
his values, of keeping communication with
relevant reference groups open and can-
did, etc. For some of the activists, it
meant his using his authority qua authority to quell the uprising. Our own conclusions concurred in part with both the
activists and those who saw him as "competent," but regardless of one's ultimate
interpretation, he was a remarkably able
and thoughtful administrator.

For example, the principal kept records of: (a) all memoranda prepared for
students, parents, and faculty; (b) let-
ters from the parent community commenting
on his performance while the movement was
most visible and active; (c) a "case study"--in parable form--which he himself
wrote about student activism in the school;
and (d) newspaper clippings on the local
and national level about activism. These
documents provided an excellent way to get
inside the principal's head and see how
his values, educational ideology, and siz-
ing up of the situation related to his behavior as educational leader. He is now
a superintendent, but left the numerous
records which were made available to us.

We supplemented this material with structured interviews of a sample of teachers
and students, looked back through local
newspapers, and studied the minutes of
Board of Education meetings to round out
as best we could what had actually been
done.

The ecological perspective became
a tremendously useful way to organize
this large amount of data and, focusing
on the educational leadership, we were
able to discuss some interesting implications for adaptive leadership in this
kind of situation. Briefly, the principle of interdependence led us to search
out the nature of the relationships between the principal and both the formal
and informal groups inside the school and
out. Inside groups included the student
government, the United Student Movement,
the "hoods" who physically opposed the
long-hairs in the Movement, etc. Outside
groups included the PTA, the school superintendent, and the general parent community. An additional concern--not always
articulated--was the interdependence between the principal's own personal values
and goals with actions mandated by the
situation. "Does he believe in what he's
doing and how he is doing it?" became an
additional focus of inquiry. The adaptation principle suggested a focus on broader norms of the school and the community.
Both content and process norms became critical in determining the outcome of the
student power movement. The bypassing of
traditional channels and the perceived
usurpation of traditional perogatives on
the part of the activists, for example,
helped alienate them from their student

peers and contrasted with the explicit and
scrupulous "going through channels" of the
principal. What the activists proposed,
in addition, did not receive significant
student support because, in essence, their
view of the school was shared by very few
other students. Regardless, this concern
with relating the process and content of
activism to broader norms was a helpful
conceptual enterprise.

The cycling of resources proved pivotal in assessing the efficacy of administrative behavior. The manner in
which he articulated the need for outside
resources relevant to the crisis, his use
of these resources in his own anticipatory
problem-solving, and his development of
constituencies inside the school and out
to function as resources to him in times
of trouble; all were paramount areas of
investigation, areas which, in our view,
generated the most fruitful implications
not only for crisis-management but for
the more general problem of institutional
development as a priority for educational
leadership. The historical perspective
suggested by the Succession principle also
provided fruitful grounds for inquiry.
The current principal had in his favor,
for example, a historical knowledge of
how the school did business through prior
experience in the school. He had taught
at the school, left to teach in a neighboring district, and was invited back to
be principal. Thus, he was a known quan-
tity to both the faculty and the community. Further, he clearly defined and adopt-
ed the anticipatory problem-solving stance
which this ecological principle suggests;
a stance made more important in public

education by the lack of institutional
means to accomplish psychosocial and policy planning.

Throughout this case study, I found
the ecological analogy helpful in thinking about how to look at the high school
as a community and, particularly, how to
focus on important aspects of the role of
principal as a part of that community.
An analogy is not a theory, nor can it
remain in the form of analogy forever.
In the quest to assess and conceptualize
communities, we must concretize the implications of this analogy in terms of
specific questions and the relation of
such variables as student-teacher interdependence and the exchange of informal
resources. However, as a basis for directing inquiry and suggesting what areas
are in need of more focused inquiry, I
found it invaluable.

These, then, are the general areas
were I have been thinking and working.
They are predicated on the assertion that
one viable definition of community psychology involves conceptual efforts in two
related areas: first, the effort to understand communities, be they defined as
neighborhoods or schools or even classrooms; second, the effort to see individual behavior in the context of an ongoing social environment which affects it
in multiple ways.

COMMUNITY PSYCHOLOGY AND THE UNIVERSITY

After leaving Stanford, I went to
Yale to work at the Psycho-Educational

Clinic as part of the academic faculty
in Psychology, where I had the opportunity to devote half my teaching load to consultation in high schools and supervision
of graduate students who, through internships, also served as school consultants.
Here was an opportunity not afforded in
postdoctoral research: namely, to start
practicing what you preach. Actually,
that phrase is not quite appropriate as
I had no integrated framework for working
as a consultant unless my role in the
"state hospital" model as "outside expert-
critic" was the model of choice. On the
levels of diagnosis, intervention, and
evaluation of change, I would not be faced
with different concerns. Yet it would
give me the opportunity to: (a) have a
prolonged and sustained relationship with
a school and school system; and (b) be
around enough to investigate informally,
yet thoroughly, the psychosocial environment of the school, its varied resources,
and its formal and informal group relationships, all from the unique perspective of help-giving consultant.

After three years of this work, I and
my coworkers have consultative experience
in several different schools and in several different roles, ranging from individual counseling—usually a diagnostic and
planning-oriented role rather than a
therapeutic one—to program creation.
Several aspects of consultation have been
particularly rewarding; and we hope to
provide a series of case studies in the
future. To give one example, let me briefly describe what Dave Todd and I call the
ecology of assessment. Hopefully this
will give a flavor of the process of trans-

lation of the ecological analogy into making choices about how to behave.

The Ecology of Assessment: The Assessment of Individual Behavior

The application of the ecological
analogy to assessment of the individual,
as we attempt it in our consultation, is
seen as related to both diagnostic assessment and decisions around intervention.
The consultant's role is both as expert
and collaborator in intervention decisions
--an assessment role which often includes
psychodiagnostic testing, though usually
around focused, circumscribed questions.
When diagnostic testing is involved, its
use as a means of educating school faculty is often coequal with its purpose of
information gathering--in short, the in-
tent is to demonstrate to a test-consci-
ous environment what such testing can and
cannot accomplish. First, let me describe
the assessment questions into which we
translate commonly arising referral questions. A primary question suggested by
the analogy is "In how many and what kinds
of settings does a given behavior occur?"
The attempt here is to isolate the context or contexts in which maladaptive behavior is reported. Second, "How many and
which of the participants in those settings express that behavior?" The greater the number and variety of persons ex-
hibiting a behavior in a particular setting and not in other settings, the more
appropriate it is to identify characteristics of the setting, rather than the
individual, which may be causative.

That is the point at which we start
when a referral comes through, be it from
teachers, guidance personnel, or administration. The primary task is to look at
the students' behavior in a number of settings (such as classes, gym, or even walk-
ing in the halls, etc.--all become foci
for understanding) to determine consist-
ency and variability. The history which
led to referral is discussed at length
with the person making the referral. Because most of our work is in "Title One"
or "Project" schools, the number of formal indigenous resources for dealing with
problem behavior is minimal and, for that
reason, only the most flagrantly disturbed students are usually referred. Usually the behavior of these students varies
from one setting to another, stemming from
an "interaction effect" with select settings rather than a "setting effect." We
also gather teacher reports of students'
behavior and often conduct short, semi-
structured interviews with the student
around how he sees his referral and his
place in the school. Thus, the thrust is
toward a life-space interview focusing on
understanding how the student operates in
different contexts. The "person in context" process is completed by more specific personological questions and, on occasion, diagnostic testing.

Another equally important thrust is
the assessment of resources for dealing
with the problems. This occurs with the
student in the short interview where he
is essentially asked to describe who the
trusted people in his social network are;
peers, teachers, a local minister, whatever. Questionnaires given to teachers

concerning classroom behavior ask about
a student's in-class friends and whether
or not the teacher has a good relationship with the student or would be willing
to develop one.

After this information gathering is
done, a meeting is held between relevant
people--often including interested teach-
ers--and the appropriate guidance counselor. The consultant attempts to summarize relevant data, and plans for intervention are made. The consultant usually declines to act as direct helper,
but offers assistance to informal help-
ers as they deal with the situation. Much
time is spent matching individual needs
with environmental circumstances, including the suggestion of altering "environments" rather than working with the student.

There are several aims of this, some
consistent with general rhetoric of consultation, some not. The first is to help
relevant school personnel think ecologic-
ally about students, to counteract the
widespread attribution of the "causes" of
behavior to intrapsychic factors only.
The second is to help teachers and guidance personnel orient themselves to a "resources" concept of people, to see the
school as a pool of formal and informal
resources ready and willing to be tapped.
Consultation is "expert" in the sense of
providing specialized skills (e.g., testing) and specialized knowledge, but also
in providing back-up and support for action plans carried out by others. An interesting outgrowth of this approach is
that, as problems become manifest and no

available resources for problem-solving
become evident, we become increasingly
aware of the needs in the school for particular kinds of programs, policies, and
personnel. One rather disturbing recent
example involved a girl in the Resource
Room--primarily a room for emotionally
and mentally retarded--who was doing well
in some regular classes at the school,
prompting us to question how she would do
totally outside the Resource Room. In
assessing her behavior and potential, we
discovered that there was no precedent
for getting out of that room; in short, no
such policy existed. Therefore, the case
went beyond recommendations about the girl
into policy implications as well, and now
formal periodic reviews occur for students
in such circumstances.

Intervention and Institutional Affiliation

One reasonable question about this
kind of consultation work emanating from
an academic institution is--baldly stated
--where's the research? It is a fair
question which relates to not only my conception of both science and research, but
one which will help focus on the last area
I want to talk about, the University as a
setting for the development of Community
Psychology. We will soon have six or
seven case studies of our work in high
schools and junior high schools over the
past three years. From these combined
documents I belive we can begin to draw
some middle-level principles about consultation as a sustained process which focuses on both people and environments. As
I believe it should be, the process of
generating hard data has had to wait for

the accumulated self-education of the
participants. Consultation is not a simple extension of the skills acquired during graduate school, but involves development of new skills and knowledge bases.
Hence, until we have a reasonable grasp
of the dimensions of the necessary skills
and knowledge, we should invest our energies in gaining the prerequisite kinds of
experiences, regardless of their potential institutional consequences. Well
documented, thoughtfully described case
studies should do wonders for the area of
psychological consultation--an area I feel
is in sore need of some sort of intellectual geritol. My academic heritage com-
pels me to emphasize that if I am still
opting for case studies 10 years from now,
I will feel like I've "copped out" on hard
thinking, but at this point I have no such
qualms.

My perception of the university as
an institution, however, leads me to believe that there may be--at this stage
of development of at least certain areas
of community psychology--a somewhat para-
lyzing tension for those of us attempting
to set this tone. Let me briefly spell
out some of my worries from the perspective of: (a) a junior faculty member;
(b) in an academic department of psychology in a university; and (c) who is part
of a clinical/community program.

COMMUNITY PSYCHOLOGY AS A
NEW CONTENT AREA

Previously, I mentioned my general
worry about the viability of community

psychology thriving in academic departments, especially when organizationally
indistinguishable from clinical psychology. My general experience at Yale is
that competent psychologists can--as individual psychologists--survive almost
anywhere. Darwin would, I am sure, agree
that some individuals have greater niche
breadth than others, but my concern is
more in the area of "institutionalizing"
community psychology. I do not know a
random sample of community psychologists,
but I have been fairly active in Division
27, the Division of Community Psychology.
Over the last three years, a better-than-
chance number of my acquaintances have
moved out of clinical areas, sometimes
out of departments altogether. Ira Iscoe
is not in the clinical area anymore. Neither is Mort Bard at CUNY or Ira Goldenberg at Harvard. Jim Kelly is Dean of an
Institute for Community Service and Public Affairs, Seymour Sarason is quartered
at the Center for the Study of Education
at Yale, Phil Mann has, I believe, opted
for a public administration position, and
among many other colleagues my own age
there is an increasing concern about being the Community Nigger. All of us have
backgrounds in clinical psychology. On
the other side, of course, are those such
as Emory Cowen who continue to "hang
tough" in clinical areas of academic departments of psychology. Still, on balance I suggest that my observations im-
ply that searching for alternate host environments for the development of the
field is in process.

While part of the explanation may
indeed lie in the personalities of those

who move away from clinical, there is, in
my opinion, a somewhat debatable "program-
environment" fit between community psychology, academic psychology, and the history
and traditions of the university. Let me
briefly outline three interdependent aspects of university-based community psychology which, I submit, make it a rather
high-risk mutant within the areas of academic psychology. These aspects deal with
the content of community psychology, the
varied methods for understanding this content, and the consequent professional
lifestyle dictated by the content. They
also provide the frame of reference for
what I see as a paramount issue for the
field, the development of professional and
scientific criteria for accountability and
competence. The mandate of the community
psychologist is to work toward the development of such criteria as the only safe-
guard against intellectual extinction and
long-term irrelevance.

In terms of content, I think it extremely important to separate--in princi-
ple--the extension of clinical activities
(based on clinical research) to new settings (essentially, what is currently defined as Community Mental Health) from the
generation of new knowledge and genuinely
different ways of behaving. Let me briefly amplify some content areas germane to
my conception of community psychology in
an effort to clarify--in terms of the content of research--this distinction.

If we start with the premise that by
semantic implication if not consensual
definition community psychology takes the
setting or community as an important level

of analysis, then several new content
areas emerge. For example, one might worry about the development, evolution, and
change of institutions or communities over
time. Seymour Sarason has initiated a
promising series of papers and a book on
one aspect of this question, the creation
of settings (Sarason, 1972): What deter-
mines the form a new setting will take,
and how do its origins relate to its evolution? A second area involves the conceptualization and assessment of human environments. This conceptualization can
provide a taxonomic, empirical, descriptive picture within which to place the
immediate context of behavior. A third
area might be the effecting of change:
strategies of intervention and planned
social change. As Chris Argyris pointed
out three years ago, our theories of intervention are crude and underdeveloped.
In my judgment, nothing has changed since
then. Equally absent, however, is a clear
picture of the interpersonal skills relevant to being a successful participant in
varied change efforts. Our experience,
for example, does not indicate that good
clinicians and good school consultants
are necessarily the same people. Regardless, this third content area mandates an
empirical examination of the conceptual
knowledge and interpersonal skills necessary for effective work in community psychology, and is based on the assumption
that substantive knowledge about environments and individuals in context must be
generated as a prelude to intervention.
Spatterings of relevant knowledge can be
found in such apparently disparate fields
as administrative science, urban planning,
and, indeed, psychology. In terms of

generating knowledge, however, clearly
there's plenty to be done. Doing it, however, brings us to the issue of methodology.

Substance and Method are Interdependent

My more cynical colleagues often in-
sist that a perennial problem within academic psychology is the insistence with
which we fit our subject matter into the
tried and true methods of the field, most
often experimental methods, of which laboratory research is seen as the paradigm.
While this paradigm has been generous to
psychology in a number of areas, those
content areas described above do not ac-
comodate well to the salient models of
our discipline. I am immensely heartened
by the writings and orientation of Harold
Raush in this general vein.

To take one example, some phenomena
such as the way in which a school utilizes
and cycles its indigenous resources during a crisis may lend itself to a case
study approach as a first approximation
to generating cogent hypotheses about community dynamics. Observation and careful
description have indeed often characterized initial scientific inquiry in many
areas. But what are the defining criteria
of such a case study? How do we know a
good case study from a bad case study and
how, in the anecdotal style characterizing
many case studies, does one distinguish
between heuristic science and good jour-
nalism? In the answers to such questions
lie some of the substantive bases on which
valid knowledge can be developed. I feel
that it is somewhat ironic to plead with

my fellow community psychologists to attend to methodology at a time when methodological nit-picking in academic psychology has served to distract some from the
pursuit of significant problems and coopted the dreams and aspirations for doing good which motivated many others; however, it is essential that we worry about
methodology if the area is to develop and
maintain intellectual respectability and
professional viability. My own lack of
professional socialization for this task
and the extremely seductive rewards of
being where the action is make this task
doubly challenging. The lack of such criteria, however, leaves one with a tremendous liability in an academic community,
the absence of defensible criteria of scientific accountability for his professional efforts. If we in universities are to
remain focused on the "out there" content
of Community Psychology, we must address
ourselves to methodology.

This stance is of particular import
for young faculty who enter this methodological thicket as novices, not as professionals with a cushion of recognized expertise. I am reminded of a discussion
involving a colleague who was one of the
designers of the early evaluations of Head
Start. Time was limited and the resultant
design and tools for analysis were less
than optimal. As I understand it, my colleague suggested that he would have been
more reluctant to commit himself to a project with such real methodological problems if he had not accrued a solid national reputation as a methodologist in
more academic pursuits. The professional
bank account of most of my youngish col-

leagues is not so flush. To my mind, however, there is no way of short-cutting
this pivotal area of learning for academically-oriented community psychologists.

Professional Lifestyle of the University-Based Community Psychologist

Thus far the assertion is twofold:
(a) that many central content areas of
community psychology are areas about which
we need to know much more, and (b) the
methodologies appropriate to the study of
these areas are either not very sophisticated or are underrepresented in current
training programs, or both. Coupled with
these is a professional lifestyle unusual
in academic traditions.

The tension implicit in this is succinctly stated by Kelly: "The adaptive
tasks of the Community Psychologist are
not to adapt to the university: his tasks
are to follow the life course of the community and to adapt to the community environment" (1970, p. 528). Taken seriously this implies a new domain of professional accountability; namely, to that
group, community, or institution where
one's professional experience and learning opportunities occur. This approach
has multiple ramifications.

First, it requires the development
over time of a relationship with a locale
which is reciprocal, collaborative, and
enduring. This expenditure of time, energy, and caring is often a prelude to
any systematic study. Thus, one demonstrates his commitment without guarantee
of even the possibility of scholarly in-

vestigation, which is a singular criterion
of the academic milieu.

In addition, the time perspective is
often concerned with phenomena which take
time to unfold and whose effects are multiple and longitudinal. Another potentially differentiating aspect lies in the
control and source of research problems
which may be generated. The process of
generating research, especially in the
area of designing interventions, often
comes as a consequence of immersion in a
particular locale and is sometimes defined by what members of the community
deem important. Immediate human needs
may supercede theoretical speculations as
an impetus for research, and this may be
a condition for the survival over time of
the community psychologist in that setting.

In sum, the professional lifestyle
of the community psychologist suggests a
series of commitments and reciprocal relationships outside the university structure which involve a redefinition of the
research relationship and the conditions
for generating knowledge. This lifestyle
is not only legitimate, but mandated by
the nature of the content of community
psychology.

THE UNIVERSITY AS NEIGHBORHOOD:
ACADEMIC PSYCHOLOGY AS HOME

Let me now make clear my bigotry
about the university as neighborhood and
academic psychology as home. One of my
blind spots in opting for an academic po-

sition was, interestingly enough, one
which is suggested as critical by the ecological analogy; namely, the historical
development of the university as an institution and the development of academic
psychology as a scientific enterprise.
As I understand it (in overly simplistic
terms), the university developed as a
place for the nourishment of thought, not
"relevance" of thought, and the primary
relationship between the university and
society is an indirect one. The influence of the university on the culture has
been seen historically as the influence
on students who, after leaving the university, made social waves through their
own careers. In this sense, the mission
of the university has never been in the
realm of action so much as enlightenment,
detachment from the immediate pressures
of the world, and debate and reflection.

Academic departments of psychology,
as I see them, nourish the same notion
of "indirect" service to mankind, and in
this are accurate reflections of the basic mission of the university. The specific frame of reference by which this
mission in psychology is judged is the
scientific enterprise, an essentially conservative one--often at the .05 or .01
level. Ad hominum appeals and resorts to
"relevance" are themselves quite irrelevant. The quality of research in academic
psychology is contingent on the dual criteria of originality and depth of ideas,
and of scientific accountability. If
there are clear rules of inference and
tested and refined methods of experiment-
ation, then it becomes possible to identify clearly good work and bad. The cre-

ative exercise generating the ideas is
then vindicated by its experimental or
empirical confirmation. In some ultimate
sense, it is the degree of scientific accountability which makes an idea credible
in academic psychology. When the criteria
of accountability are fuzzy, the originality and depth of ideas behind the research is more open to question.

In many areas, academic psychology
has developed an elaborate and increasingly refined methodological history.
When a field such as experimental social
psychology has been around long enough to
have what was originally an artifact (e.g.,
experimenter bias) become a well-investi-
gated phenomenon in its own right, that's
a substantial developmental history. My
contention is that the methods appropriate
to study in community psychology do not
have this fortunate history of increasing
sophistication and refinement. This
places community psychology, as a new
field with new problems requiring new
ways of study, at an inherent disadvant-
age in an academic community governed by
criteria of accountability which, in many
areas, have a significant history. In
addition, in the process--the necessary
process--of our own self-education, many
of us have gotten caught up in the act of
doing, with the magical fantasy that either doing would suffice, or that combin-
ing doing and thinking were not extremely
trying tasks. The academic culture is a
thinking, not a doing, culture, so much
so that it often judges as suspect the
mere activity of doing even if it is the
best way to learn how to think well about
something.

I firmly believe in the values of
conception, of data gathering, and of research in general, and I think that community psychology needs this focus for its
own development. To the extent that my
portrayal of the interdependence of content, method, and professional lifestyle
of the academically-oriented community
psychologist mirrors reality, however, I
believe there is a real tension between
the traditions of the university and the
current struggles and aspirations of the
evolving domains of community psychology.
Dealing with this tension in a creative
and integrating rather than alienating
and self-defeating way seems to me to be
a paramount question for both universities
and community psychologists. I am not at
all certain about what the varied outcomes
might look like.

I also have some qualms about seeing
community psychology as a subspecialty of
clinical psychology, although this is the
clear structural implication of, say, ad-
vertising for a community psychologist to
join one's clinical area. Regardless of
current practice, I believe that, on a
conceptual level, such a stance is inap-
propriate, unless one defines community
psychology as community mental health.
The assumptions about the level of analysis of behavior, indeed assumptions about
the nature of man, are different enough
to merit independent status. I've seen
too many friends and colleagues try to
straddle the fence, becoming hyphenated
psychologists to appease both their interests and the host environment. Indeed,
the very image of straddling fences is
good enough to suggest significant psy-

chic discomfort.

I am neither suggesting a rejection
of clinical training nor suggesting that
existing clinical roles cannot be stretch-
ed to include significant doses of environmental intervention. Indeed, my own
competencies--whatever they may be--have
been heavily influenced by my own clinical
training. However, I believe that in addition to the elaboration of the clinical
role in a more "community-oriented" direction, separate efforts are needed to develop new roles and new knowledge not necessarily linked to clinical assumptions.
As a result of my own experience, I feel
both a need and an obligation to create
a place and a program which minimize the
amount of reeducation one must do upon
leaving.

One final worry is worth mentioning
along these general lines: that is the
potentially intimidating effect on students in dealing with this institutional
tension. At my own university, more than
one student has said, either directly or
covertly, that he is interested in my pursuits but feels a need to "play it safe"
until he gets his degree. Certainly there
are exceptions to this, both in terms of
the independence of students and in the
perceived severity of the departmental
press, but the phenomenon, for whatever
reasons, is a real one representing, in my
judgment, an unconscionable compromise.

Robert Nisbet has suggested that the
university is better suited to the refinement and elaboration of an established
field than to the creation of a new one.

I worry that what I see as necessary conditions, conditions of experiential learning, of teaching ourselves new fields, of
community accountability, of field activity, and of consequent methodological and
conceptual vagueness are too antithetical
to academic psychology at this point in
time. This is especially worrisome, I
fear, as Federal policies cause training
grants to terminate. Since World War II,
clinical psychology has subsisted primarily on federal funds, funds which Nisbet
eloquently argues have coopted the basic
mission of the university. What happens
now that the gravy train is leaving will
be interesting to observe and be part of.
Fields which attempt to blend action with
reflection are seldom core components of
the university and within departments of
psychology clinical psychology is not often core. I cannot see this as accidental.

CURRENT AND FUTURE TASKS

There are, however, areas where community psychology must develop regardless
of the institutional context in which it
exists. First there is a tremendous need
to develop a series of intellectual bases
for different areas of community psychology and to nurture methodological traditions to generate knowledge which is both
pragmatic and valid. Second, I think it
is important to think about alternative
host environments for the development of
differing community psychology competencies. Those of us in academic settings
need to weigh the history of our particular academic culture--its traditions and
prospects for the future--against our de-

finition of the lifestyle demands of the
community psychologist.   Third, there is
a need to develop a local and national
identity with other community psychologists and professionals in related areas.
I've gotten a good deal of pleasure working in Division 27, and it has been personally important to see it as a reference group.   It is also frustrating and
time-consuming; however, I'm concerned
that so many people interested in community psychology have had such a hard time
generating a sense of community and an
appreciation for the task at hand.   In
the formative years of any venture, an
inordinate amount of energy is required
to get it off the ground.   I see it as
a struggle for the Division to get itself
together.   A friend who is a Washington,
D.C., psychoanalyst and on a review committee which visits Institutes to evaluate the quality of analytic training, recently remarked how curious it was that
people who spend their lives understanding others had so many organizational problems.   That didn't seem silly to me because I don't see analytic theory--as applied to individuals--as being particularly predictive of organizational behavior.
To the degree that professionals in community psychology do the same thing, however, we're in trouble.

In conclusion, it has been a tremendously gratifying experience sharing with
you--hopefully in the spirit of this colloquium series--my own work and worries
about community psychology.   I have not
approached this task as one might approach
a scholarly colloquium, and I am grateful
to Stu Golann for removing those constraints.

What I have attempted to do is convey the flavor of my own efforts to define a viable professional lifestyle in the evolving area of community psychology. Clearly any definitive resolution lies in the future. Still, as I reflect on my own education, I keep being reminded of a line from one of my favorite songs: "the treasure's not the taking, it's the loving of the game."

ACKNOWLEDGMENT

The author wishes to thank Maryrose Carew and Carol Hammond for their editorial help with earlier drafts of the manuscript.

REFERENCES

Carew, M. Perceived self-environment similarity and satisfaction in two age levels of truant and regular high school students. Yale University, 1973, mimeo.

Cooper, L. Staff attitudes about ideal wards before and after program change. Journal of Community Psychology, 1973, 1, 82-84.

Endler, N. S., & Hunt, J. S-R inventories of hostility and comparisons of proportions of variance from persons, responses, and situations for hostility and anxiousness. Journal of Personality and Social Psychology, 1968, 9, 309-315.

Highbee, K. L., & Wells, M. G. Some research trends in social psychology during the 1960's. *American Psychologist*, 1972, *27*, 963-966.

Katz, D., & Kahn, R. *Social psychology of organizations*. New York: Wiley, 1966.

Kaufman, B. *Up the down staircase*. Englewood Cliffs, N.J.: Prentice-Hall, 1965.

Kelly, J. G. Antidotes for arrogance: Training for community psychology. *American Psychologist*, 1970, *25*, 524-531.

Miles, M. B. Some properties of schools as social systems. In G. Watson (Ed.) *Change in school systems*. Washington, D.C.: National Training Lab, NEA, 1967.

Moos, R. H., & Trickett, E. J. *Classroom environment scale manual*. Palo Alto, Calif.: Consulting Psychologists Press, 1973 (in press).

Ochberg, F. M., & Trickett, E. J. Administrative responses to racial tensions in a high school. *Community Mental Health Journal*, 1970, *6*, 470-483.

Pierce, W. D., Trickett, E. J., & Moos, R. H. Changing ward atmosphere through staff discussion of the perceived ward environment. *Archives of General Psychiatry*, 1972, *26*, 35-41.

Raush, H. L., Dittman, A. T., & Taylor, T. T. Person, setting and change in social interaction. *Human Relations*, 1959, *12*, 361-378. (a)

Raush, H. L., Dittman, A. T., & Taylor, T. T. The interpersonal behavior of children in residential treatment. Journal of Abnormal and Social Psychology, 1959, 58, 9-26. (b)

Sarason, S. B. The creation of settings and the future societies. San Francisco: Jossey-Bass, 1972.

Schneider, B. The perception of organizational climate: The customer's view. Unpublished manuscript, University of Maryland, 1972.

Stern, G. People in context. New York: Wylie Press, 1970.

Trickett, E. J., Kelly, J. G., & Todd, D. M. The social environment of the high school: Guidelines for individual change and organizational development. In S. Golann & C. Eisendorfer (Eds.) Handbook of community mental health. New York: Appleton-Century-Crofts, 1972, 331-401.

Trickett, E. J., & Moos, R. H. Generality and specificity of student reactions in high school classrooms. Adolescence, 1970, 20, 373-390.

Trickett, E. J., & Moos, R. H. Satisfaction with the correctional institution environment: An instance of perceived self-environment similarity. Journal of Personality, 1972, 40(1), 75-87.

Trickett, E. J., & Moos, R. H. Social environment of junior high and high school classrooms. Journal of Educational <u>Psychology</u>, 1973, <u>65</u>(1), 93-102.

Trickett, E. J., & Ochberg, F. D.   The ecology of educational leadership: A case study of student activism and administrative coping.   Yale University, 1973. (mimeo)

Trickett, E. J., & Todd, D. M.   The assessment of the high school culture: An ecological perspective. <u>Theory</u> <u>into</u> <u>Practice</u>, 1972, <u>11</u>, 28-37.

5. BECOMING A COMMUNITY PSYCHOLOGIST

Ira Iscoe

I was pleased to have been invited
as one of the speakers in the Community
Psychology Series. I have had great respect for the program at the University
of Massachusetts and I have every confidence that it will continue to grow and
address itself to the salient problems
facing community psychology today. I
understood that I was supposed to hold
forth for about an hour or so and then
answer questions. I was also asked to
give to the best of my ability some background of how I got into community psychology and finally describe some of the
things that I am doing or thinking about
doing.

In some ways I have a little bit of
trepidation in tracing before graduate
students how I got into community psychology. Most of us so-called Senior People
in the field certainly didn't get into it
by the paths by which you are getting into it. In many ways our age is one in
which there is little relevant knowledge
of the past to be applied to the present.

So bear with me and if you see some paral-
lels or some possibilities all the better. If not, then at least I will have
enjoyed the reminiscing.

In thinking about what I was going
to talk about, I had to go over a lot of
territory trying to find out how I got
into the area. I have spent a lot of
time getting here. I am 52 years of age.
I graduated in 1951 from UCLA in the area
of child clinical. I probably was better
trained than most of the clinicians today. I had extremely good training and
projective techniques under Bruno Kleopfer and I was pretty sure that I was going to work with kids and I did. I was
assistant to Grace M. Frenald and to El-
len B. Sullivan and to the whole bash
down there at the clinical school. I
soon became an expert in reading disabilities, and indeed Frenald on her death
bed made me promise that I would do the
definitive work on why reading disabilities occurred so frequently in boys.
It's, as you know, a ratio of about 6 or
7 to 1. I didn't pursue that work, un-
fortunately, and incidentally, the definitive work is still to be done. There
was the UCLA clinic at which I did part
of my internship and there, too, I got a
lot of experience with children. Fannie
Montalto (since deceased) was a very excellent child therapy supervisor. I also
did a lot of volunteer work at various
places in and around Los Angeles. Then,
as now, it was important to really go out
and get some of the experience on your own
and not to wait for the department or your
professors to do it for you. I was perhaps more fortunate than most in that I

had some professors very much interested
in me. They made enormous demands on my
time yet they provided me with all sorts
of experiences and really helped to ma-
ture me as a graduate student in rather
short order. In my time, as in the present, there were the usual departmental
politics and I went through an agonizing
period with the loyalty oath conflict at
the University of California. I became
appreciative of how careful a graduate
student had to be within a department and
I was also very admiring of the courage
displayed by some of my professors in
their resistance to the loyalty oath. Incidentally, the whole thing was soon thrown
out by the California Supreme Court.

In terms of support, I had, I guess,
one of the first U. S. Public Health fel-
lowships awarded in fellowshipery. This
was awarded in 1949 and this, plus being
a bigshot in the clinical school and tutoring kids who had reading disability,
made graduate school from time to time a
rather well paying occupation. I left
eventually to come to Texas in 1951 at
the salary of $3900 for 9 months, some-
what of a comedown for a hot-shot child
clinician, but it was close to the going
rate at that time. Why did I go to Texas?
Actually, I went there for only a year.
There were other offers that hadn't quite
come through. One or two of my mentors
at Texas pointed out that Carl M. Dallen-
bach had moved from Cornell to establish
a department there and that Wayne Holtz-
man had just arrived the year before and
that Harry Helson was also going to join
the staff. It seemed like a good place
to start. In Texas, my job was to help

develop the clinical program and to get
it approved. Although I had had good experience with children and adults and rather good training in psychoanalysis
(plus a didactic personal analysis) I
didn't feel very competent. Nevertheless,
we did develop the program and it was approved. Remember now that I had been
trained in the "psychic primacy" approach
in which early impressions and personality
development were most important. As far
as the problems of the world were concerned, as soon as more therapists were put
out in my likeness we'd get to them.
There was some vague talk about social
workers and the environment, but this was
secondary. The important thing was the
development of the person and how he perceived the world. The jurisdictional dis-
putes about who should "do" psychotherapy
were then in full bloom, so to speak, and
I was, of course, of the school that only
Ph.D. level psychologists should be allowed to administer the sacrament of psychotherapy. I was, however, even then
convinced that the most a Ph.D. granted
you as far as clinical work was concerned
was really more confidence to say you
didn't know. This, of course, is a very
important advantage. As graduate students,
as you know, on cue you are supposed to
get into certain things and to be knowledgeable. You hardly ever admit that
you don't know. Once you get your degree,
there are a lot of other guys that don't
know, and what's more, you can also say,
"If you give me some money, I'll research
the area." I mention this because I am
convinced that it is only after one leaves
graduate school that one really begins to
learn. The groundword is laid in graduate

school. In looking back I think I was
very fortunate. I had some awfully good
mentors in graduate school as I have said.
In fact, my coming to Texas was due to advice of some professors.

Austin, Texas, allowed for the expansion of my clinical skills. There were
many institutional and private facilities
which had never had a child clinical psychologist near them. I volunteered for a
number of situations and at numerous times
in the first few years I did the psycholo-
gicals at the Cerebral Palsy Center. I
acted for no pay as Chief Psychologist at
Austin State Hospital. I did the work at
the Juvenile Court and also in the County
Jail. Here, too, I didn't realize it at
first, but I was picking up a tremendous
amount of experience in the community. I
also got to know the people in the school
pretty well. There were no psychological
services in the Austin School System to
speak of in 1951 and this was a not in-
considerable system, possessing at that
time over 35,000 students. I learned to
work with many of the problems that teachers presented and I began to appreciate
the enormous complexity that goes into
financing and running a school system. I
became very good friends with the school
superintendent and, for that matter, most
of the members of the school board. I
guess here is where I laid the basis for
some of my later interest in mental health
consultation.

From time to time I have regretted
not having had more work in education. It
might have facilitated easier acceptance
within public school systems, and as sort

of a flashback, I do recall that while
at UCLA I did try to combine a major of
education and psychology. No Way! The
psychology building was right across from
the education building. One day one of
my mentors saw me coming out of the education building and sneered appropriately. I was given to understand that education and psychology were never to come
together as long as this particular men-
tor was alive. I also, as a teaching assistant, used to participate in the yearly summer slaughter of teachers who had
to take a course or two in psychology.
Looking back at it, we certainly commit-
ted some atrocities on the poor teachers,
forcing them to learn learning theory all
on rats and mostly Hullian, while the poor
creatures had innocently stepped in to
learn something about human behavior.

While I also did a lot of teaching
at Texas, I was a clinician and we did
open a child clinic in our new building.
Incidentally Mezes Hall, which opened
about 1953, was the first building in the
United States planned and built entirely
for psychology. At its dedication the
upper crust of psychology were present
and the august Society of Experimental-
ists honored it by holding probably its
first and only meeting ever held in the
Southwest. Looking back at it, I did like
my clinical work. Even today I love to
look at batteries of tests and once a year
I do a blind Rorschach for the graduate
students in clinical (a little beer in
me helps). All I ask is the age and sex
of the person and I do pretty well indeed.
Naturally, I think the content analysis
of the Rorschach is valid for me. I can't

prove it, but more often than not I get
some awfully good insights about the personality of the person. I also respect
better constructed, from a psychometric
point of view, instruments like the WISC
and the WAIS. Despite attacks on them
they are valid instruments for certain
purposes and if, for example, you get an
IQ of 120 and a student is failing in
school, you do not say that the test is
wrong. You ask a better question: "What
is it that permits a person with an IQ
in this level to blow it in school?"
This does signify some problems.

I have often asked myself where my
interest in community first started. I
suppose most productive community mental
healthers and community psychologists are
pretty astute connivers and bargainers.
I am not necessarily a politician, but
somehow I have learned power distributions
and the sharing of goals. In addition,
my own background in a Jewish family presented understandably a high achievement
motivation. Contrary to some of the present approaches, we Jewish boys growing
up in Montreal, Canada, never expected a
break and never hoped to get by with less.
You knew that you weren't going to make it
and your Yiddish momma never ceased re-
minding you that it was a cruel world out
there and that the Goyim were not going
to allow you any leeway for errors. Education was a way out of the ghetto. Jewish boys went into McGill or else into
business. As a kid in school you began
to learn the forces in the community and
where you fit in. In grade school I was
one of three Jewish kids in the entire
school. Some of you will recognize that

in Quebec at that time there were two
school systems, namely one run by the Protestant Board of School Commissioners and
the other one run by the Catholic Commissioners. If you were Jewish you went to
the Protestant school unless there wasn't
one, in which case you went to the Catholic school. For two years I went to a
Catholic school in a small town north of
Montreal and everything was really fine
because it was obvious that I would soon
be converted. I could say mass and Pater
Nosters with the best of them and I'm sure
that Orthodox Hebrew chants and the Latin
hymns had very much in common, in terms
of melodies. I soon learned that you had
different relationships with Protestant
kids than you did with Catholics. With
the Catholic kids we'd joke around. They
were openly antisemitic. They kidded us,
and sometimes not kidded us, about being
Jewish and we replied with obscenities
against nuns, priests, and their sexual
relationships, etc. Eventually sort of
a truce was reached, but you learned to
stand your ground and fight. With the
Protestants it was different. When a
Protestant school was opened, I was transferred to it. The Protestants had it over
both Jews and Catholics economically. The
Catholics were even worse off than the
Jews were. The Protestants had power.
They too were a numerical minority amongst
the French Canadians, but they had control
of most of the finances. You pretty soon
learned about power distributions and you
learned pretty soon to find your way
through the system. Sometimes you found
that you could mediate quarrels between
the French Canadian kids and the Catholic
kids. Many times I was impressed with

how friendly we could all be under certain situations and how quickly we could
revert to savagery under various types
of threats and sometimes parental influence. I might recite one incident which
can show you that antisemetic French
Canadian boys still have need for a Jewish boy. In a town during my adolescence,
there was only one drug store. The drives
and needs of adolescence, of course, are
well known to at least the graduate students in this room and the art and repertoire of contraceptive devices was not as
extensive as it is now. My Catholic
friends were always afraid to buy contra-
ceptives lest the druggist report them to
their parents. If a Jewish boy bought
them it was OK, and after all, even for
a religious Catholic, money was money.
I think the druggist really admired me.
After all it wasn't every adolescent that
would go and buy six to eight boxes of
Trojans at one time.

I took this diversion because I feel
that just like therapy, many of the experiences that a person has before graduate school in many ways equip him for
certain types of functions. Perhaps graduate school helps round out these experiences, or adds a certain depth to them.
At any rate, I did learn how to survive
in the community without really being
known as such. In Texas, quite naturally, I got involved in a variety of community activities. I was not a joiner in
the convivial sense of the word, but I
had the conviction, since strengthened,
that it was important to know organizations and how they related to each other.
Bear in mind that I belonged to such or-

ganizations as the Texas Association of
Mental Health and the Austin Travis County Juvenile Court. Both of these were
not exactly traditional places for a psychologist. Why did I do this? I really
couldn't say. I liked my teaching. I
taught clinical work. I supervised and
I actually turned out some awfully fine
students. It had become clear to me that
clinical psychology was going to change.
It was going to change because although
it was very comfortable for a psychologist
to pick up casualties of social systems,
it was obvious that some day some of us
would have to walk up-stream and find out
what was pushing all these casualties into the river. Social systems and their
influence on behavior had not been stressed much, if at all, in all my training.
Even in the area of child clinical, family therapy had not yet arrived on the
scene. Children would not be seen at our
Community Guidance Center unless their
parents were also in treatment and we
really picked only the best risks and paid
virtually no attention to the lower socioeconomic classes.

However, being a clinician in a psychology department rapidly gaining in
prestige can be a dangerous thing. Although I worked enormously hard as a clinician and worked in the community, very
little reward and recognition was forth-
coming. It became clear that I would have
to be better certified. I played the usual games: Research grants in the late
'50's and most of the '60's were easy to
come by. I did research on conformity in
children and in mental retardation. I
did this frankly because I was interested,

but also because it was what paid off in
a department. I enjoyed working with
Harold Stevenson who came to Texas a year
after I did and it was gratifying to see
a superb learning theorist like Stevenson
apply theoretical issues to mental retardation. Incidentally, Ed Zigler was also
a student in Texas and later on James
Kelly as well.

     With publications came some increas-
ing recognition and tenure as an Associate Professor and finally a Professor-
ship. From about 1951-1960, let us say
about 9 years, I enjoyed my work, but as
I said, I became convinced that I was being stifled in the clinical program and
could go no further. It's true that I
branched out into groups, started into
various types of family therapy, but I
really wanted to go into what was best
described then as community mental health.
I looked around and was fortunate enough
to get a senior stipend from NIH in order
to attend Gerald Caplan's community mental
health training program. When the history
of community mental health and community
psychology is written, the contributions
of Caplan and Lindemann will be recognized.
The program, of course, had a lot of de-
fects, but it did bring public health and
crisis concepts and mental health concepts
together. I had a wonderful year and I
went back to Texas in 1961 after the year
at Harvard. I'm not sure why I did it.
I had other offers, but my family and I
had grown to like Texas tremendously.

     I was disappointed when I got back
to Texas. The entire clinical program was
still pretty much a traditional one and

there was fear of offering me the Directorship of the clinical program lest I
get into that community mental health bit.
This was pretty much, however, a reflection of the times. There was no impetus
as yet for community mental health, this
being 1961. As an example of psychology's
indifference, while at the school of public health a former student of mine, Kent
Miller, now at Florida State University,
and I, worked on an article entitled "The
Concept of Crisis and its Implications
for Mental Health" (1963). It was then
the definitive article in the field. I
still think it is. It finally saw the
light of day in 1963, but not in any psychology journal. The Journal of Abnormal
and Social Psychology thought it was not
sufficiently empirical. The Psychological
Bulletin thought it was great, but it was
not a bulletin article. The Review turned
up its nose. The Journal of Consulting
Psychology didn't think its readers were
ready, etc. The Journal of Social Psychology also said no. It finally saw the
light of day in Human Organization, the
journal of the Society of Applied Anthro-
pology. Notions about a crisis, dealing
effectively with problems within crisis,
increasing the coping skills of human beings, and the need to consider properly
timed interventions were still pretty much
out in left field for psychology.

At any rate, I stayed on at Texas,
considering some other places, working
slowly and somewhat despairingly towards
a community mental health program. A
change in chairmanship gave me some encouragement and the Swampscott Conference
(Boston) in 1965 will be viewed as a turn-

ing point. The Conference, as most of
you know, was called to consider the education of clinical psychologists in community mental health. Most, if not all,
of the psychologists who attended the
conference were very accomplished and successful. Most of us had achieved diplo-
mates and were doing pretty well in the
clinical field. When we needed a little
extra money, we shot a diagnostic battery
or two. You could always test for a psychiatrist who marvelled at your acumen.

Why did the assembled group unani-
mously agree on the term community psychology? I think most of us recognized that
psychology would have to become more responsive to environmental pressures. We
recognized dimly that there were a lot of
things stirring. Some of you will recall
that the Joint Commission on Mental Illness and Health (1960) had recommended
sweeping changes, plus a hint that the
community ought to become more involved.
At any rate, community psychology emerged
and, of course, is still being attacked
for lack of clear definition, for blur-
ring of roles, and the like. One of the
favorite ways to slash a discipline or a
person apart in academia is to pin him to
the wall definitionally. I would advise
community psychologists not to get caught
in this bind. There are other so-called
more "substantive" areas in psychology
that still have the dickens of a time defining what they are about. Community
psychology deals with very complicated issues. It is not even yet 10 years old
and it should not panic.

It was pretty obvious to the conference that there would have to be some curriculum changes in order to equip psychologists for working in communities, but no firm recommendations were made. In fact, the conference showed its wisdom by not trying to make any suggestions to departments. Many of us knew that we were stepping into an area in which we had no professional training and the model of clinical psychology as one part of community mental health which in turn was one part of community psychology had different implications than the model of community psychology as part of community mental health which was part of clinical psychology. There is little to be gained even today by arguing. I, however, do hold that community psychology is a much broader undertaking than either community mental health or clinical psychology. There was some general agreement that we had to move the laboratory of the university to the laboratory of the community. This of course found many psychologists unprepared. It is interesting to note, for example, that the late Martin Luther King in his last public address, which was to the American Psychological Association, called upon American psychology to lend its skills in the solution of the race problems of America. He received a standing ovation and nothing much happened. American psychology wasn't prepared to start dealing with the problem. It's very difficult to leave the laboratory of the university with its predictabilities (and its difficulties) for the unknown forces and power in a community where the reception is not likely to be too friendly. However, if knowledge were to be

gained and eventually tested, it was apparent that it would have to be tested
in the community.

The knowledge base for clinical as
well as community psychology had to be ex-
panded. It seemed to me at that time that
there were a variety of research findings
that could be applied to the problems facing community psychology. Why this knowledge was not applied is, of course, a
different story. I might add that not
being ready when we could have been cost
us a great deal in terms of progress and
support. The advent of the new federalism with general and special revenue-shar-
ing now finds us not really prepared to
ask for our share. I have frequently said
that the knowledge base of psychology was
hindered in that many of the social ex-
periments during the Kennedy and Johnson
years were lauched without any research
provisions by psychologists and behavioral
scientists. We were lucky, however, in
that psychologists like Ed Ziegler were
able to do at least something in Project
Head Start and in the Day Care movement.
From this we have gained an immense amount
of knowledge calling for a reconsideration
of some of our more fundamental approaches.

There were, of course, some other
constraining factors. Psychology departments were "fat." They were glutted with
grants and support from other sources.
Communities in the '60's were in a rapid
state of flux and most psychology departments in prestigious universities, as indeed the universities themselves, maintained quite a separation from the community. The Community Mental Health Faci-

lities Act was passed in 1963 and soon
the community mental health centers were
beginning to gain momentum to the extent
that even today with the restrictions imposed by the Nixon administration the community mental health centers appear pretty definitely to be a major force in the
delivery of mental health and human services in America.

I want to call your attention to an
interesting phenomenon. When a new social experiment starts in a community it
is "behind the gun" so to speak and has
to succeed. It's OK for industry to plod
along with the best engineers and to invest half a billion dollars in a plane
that won't go off the ground, or if it
does go off the ground, crashes with un-
nerving frequency. That's apparently OK.
It's back to the drawing boards and cor-
rect the errors. Behavioral science ex-
periments--ah, well that's another story!
"You screwed up. I told you. I told you
it was all no good." And the experiment
is put down as a failure and once again
the high and the mighty indicate that communities and particularly the disadvant-
aged in communities are intransigent, up
to no good, unmotivated, undesiring of a
better life, happy in the slums, etc. I
might at this point say that a good community psychologist recognizes that whenever efforts are extended for one part of
the community they are called charity and
welfare. When these same efforts are extended to industry or to agriculture they
are called subsidy. When you get to add-
ing up the various types of subsidies,
you find that they are almost equal to the
amount spent in charity.

There were some other barriers to
working in the community. For instance,
when psychologists entered schools as
consultants they knew very little about
school systems and frequently "promised
to walk on water." The school people knew
very well that the local bad-acting child
was a problem beyond the ability of the
psychologist to solve. The fact that the
psychologist was naive enough to think
that he could solve the problems, or change
the school system, or conspire with one or
two teachers in order to "improve upon
things" indicates the level of his naive-
te. Little old teachers could easily take
psychologists down the primrose path.
Much the same might be said for the community mental health center. Of course
community psychologists goofed in them at
the beginning because they brought with
them a series of armaments and maneuvers
that were not suited to the community
needs. They basically applied so-called
medical models. In a tremendously interesting study by Bloom (1969) of innovative
mental health centers, he found that psychologists were helping redesign environments, they were writing grants, they were
training paraprofessionals, they were consulting to day care and human service programs and they had been trained for none
of this. However, in most of these programs good things were happening. In an
interesting article Warren (1971) pointed
out the dilemmas of the psychologist in
a model cities program. Even in the area
of research it was becoming apparent that
the training of the psychologist in more
classical analysis of variance designs
was impeding his research possibilities.
Going into communities with analysis of

variance designs does violence to the type
of research setting you are in. It became
apparent, therefore, that unobtrusive measures, multivariate analysis, and some of
the designs by Campbell and Stanley (1963)
were much more appropriate. In most
cases, however, clinical psychologists and
community mental health psychologists were
ignorant of these procedures.

I mentioned previously the difficulties psychologists were having in communities and I implied that our mode of entry was basically through community mental
health centers. This is still the case.
Community mental health centers have taken
root. For the first time in the United
States, in a relatively short period of
time at that, mental health has become
part of public financing. No matter what
the cutbacks are going to be, mental health
centers have obtained a toe-hold and will
not be phased out. They have opened a very
exciting base for psychologists--a very
important one indeed. It may be that
eventually they will be fused with human
service centers or mental health may become part of health delivery systems.
Community psychology can maintain its
growing identity if it will not get involved in traditional services, but begin
to understand the problems of the communities that are being served.

In my own county of Travis in Austin,
Texas, we have what might be described as
a fairly conservative community. There
are a lot of rednecks in the surrounding
areas and mental health is for "kooks."
Nevertheless, last year the City Council
put $130,000 into community mental health,

which is $130,000 more than they put in
four years ago. The county puts in $50,-
000, which is $50,000 more than it put in
three years ago. That's $180,00 as a
base. Not the greatest amount I admit,
but then the state puts in about one-half
million which is state money as opposed
to federal money. This is a new base on
which psychologists should operate, and
especially with the growing concern about
evaluation of services. I will make the
categorical statement that unless psychologists begin thinking of ways of evaluating services, the boys in the account-
ing office will start doing it for us.

In the rapid growth of community mental health centers, new types of manpower
have grown up and the time to evaluate
their efficacy is close at hand. I particularly worry about some of the so-called specialities that have arisen without
any theoretical basis and in some ways as
a response to the anxieties of communities. I, to this day, do not know what
a drug counselor does different from a
counselor of alcoholism or for that matter a therapist. Maybe it's part of the
fuzziness of the areas I have spoken about,
but nevertheless, some shakedown is coming. The increased sophistication of the
consumer will call for his inclusion in
the planning and delivery of service.
This is part of the collapse of boundaries and most of us know that the boun-
dary between the university and the community has become quite blurred. The
university has invaded the community and
the community has invaded the university
and the recent vote of the 18-year-olds
means that students will more than ever

influence the politics of communities and,
I am quite sure, vice versa. Rather than
cause for alarm it should be cause for
some sober thought and some excitement.
Perhaps combinations of resources can be
put together in a much more effective way.
To achieve this combination of resources
is a challenge to the community psychologist and begins to focus on one of the
main things that I have been concerned
about, namely the consequences of change.
I'd like to go a little further into this.

In my day and now in the days of increasing emphasis on the treatment of the
mentally ill in the community, the demise
of the mental hospitals as we know them
is pretty well assured. The state of California has closed down all but two of
its hospitals. This should be cause for
joy; the bastille has fallen. But presumably all of the nasty homes that have
sprung up will be the mental hospitals of
the future and the day care centers set
up in community health centers will be
the sanctuary for the chronic patient.
I'm not quite so sure that this is an improvement over the mental hospitals. Mrs.
O'Grady's Shady Rest Home may be a crueler
place than a state hospital. At least in
the state hospital you could have access
and make demands, or at least demand access. I'm not sure Mrs. O'Grady is going
to allow volunteers to come in. It will
be an interesting thing to follow. As a
matter of fact, I'm quite sure that Mrs.
O'Grady will stand on her rights as a private organization and tell community psychologists, psychiatrists, and other in-
quisitive people to stay the hell out of
her place. We see here a blending of a

variety of forces. Rest homes spring up
because there is a population to look after and some money to be made. They will,
of course, support the community mental
health movement and they will win because
mental hospitals have not developed their
lobby and it's too late now to start. A
viable community mental health center
should have a portion of its resources
invested in the assessment of the living
conditions of the population or populations it serves. It is only by ecologi-
cally-oriented long-range studies of the
patient returned from the mental hospital
that we will be able to say something definitive about his movement in the community, what resources he uses and doesn't
use, and perhaps candidly face the fact
that certain forms of mental illness,
given what we now know, do not respond to
community care much differently than hospital care. It may very well be that the
chronic schizophrenic over 40 is best kept
clean, comfortable, and schizophrenic,
and that scarce resources should not be
spent on ineffective treatment programs.

In thinking about the development of
community psychology and how I got into
it, I've recognized that we do have to
have some discipline and some conceptual
basics. As far as I'm concerned, the
great majority of departments of psychology today are not broad enough to offer
the students the wide range of academic
and experiential bases that they will need
in the community. This type of approach
raises all sorts of problems. We have
seen the difficulties that clinical psychology has had within departments of
psychology, particularly prestigious de-

partments. A separate community psychology or a separate community mental health
program raises all sorts of further problems. I simply don't want community students to have to take all the stuff that
clinical students have to. I feel that
something has got to give in community
psychology training and I for one am willing to go on record as saying that courses
in community development and mental health
consultation are as difficult to learn as
courses in basic psychology, including
animal learning. I wish to turn out a
new breed of students who, of course, will
be cognizant of some clinical aspects of
human behavior, but who will be most interested in the design, delivery, and evaluation of services to human beings. That's
where we are. There may be people who
really want to deliver the services. In
this case, I think we ought to give them
a special clinical background. For myself, I would like all students to have
some form of experience in therapy. Cy-
nic that I am, I'm not sure that all the
people just dying to get into community
psychology are really all that well put
together. It's the same suspicion that
I have had of people who have gone into
learning or personality, all the time
knocking clinical psychology. I have been
fascinated to see how many of these people five years later wind up by taking
their post-doctorals in clinical. Is it
that they have seen the light so to speak,
or were they always interested in clinical
and couldn't admit it? If you are a clinician, you can ask the question, "Why is
that guy knocking so much on other people's professions and interests?" You
know that any person who has got to make

a living by killing somebody else is really in trouble. I would really like then
a more balanced community psychologist.
I'd like him to know where his head is
and one of the ways of doing this is for
him to work with a somewhat traditional
therapist to get some of his own motivations cleared up. Incidentally, lest I
have conveyed the impression that I am
antitherapy, let me clear this up at this
point. I believe that a broad therapeutic experience in terms of human growth
is a very valuable one. Whether therapy
helps neuroses or not, I'm not sure. However, a therapeutic relationship can be,
I am convinced, of great value in helping
the human being sort out his motivations
and values. For this reason I would re-
serve psychotherapy for those persons who
will be involved in the motivations of
others. Community psychologists certainly fall into this group.

One of my other objections to current training of community psychologists,
especially within clinical psychology contexts, is that departments are unwilling
to give credit for the enormous amount of
supervision that it takes to develop a
good community psychologist. For example,
one of the great thrusts in community psychology today is consultation activities.
It's one thing to foul up a client or a
group; it's another to carry out or recommend activities that have the potential
of fouling up an entire system. One bad
afternoon can ruin a relationship that has
been built up for many years. This has
actually happened to me in my relationship
to a small public school system when a
consultant went much too fast and was much

too threatening to the teachers and the
superintendent. For this reason I sometimes despair whether good community psychology programs can emerge out of an arts
and science context. On the other hand,
within a university setting there are an
enormous amount of resources and a good
community psychology program takes advantage of the resources that are available
besides developing those that are needed.
As the pressures on universities have
grown, they have not shown the adaptabi-
lity that a devoted academician like myself would expect. Instead of multidisciplinary approaches, they have exerted
increased territorialities. This makes
it most unlikely that community psychology programs will be able to grow and
prosper in their current settings.

We should also keep in mind that many
prestigious psychology departments arrive
at their present condition under a formula
of rigid research training and isolation
from community settings. Presently there
is no reward to make them change this direction. On the other hand, more "hungry"
university settings may exhibit the flexi-
bility and the breadth of thought to produce a top-level community psychology program. For the moment I fear, or at least
I feel, that professional schools may be
the most suitable places for community
psychology training. I don't say this
with a lot of joy because I have a lot of
reservations about professional schools
and I wonder about their devotion or commitment to the fostering of genuine research. I think they make a lot of pious
statements in that direction, but I do not
as yet see the commitment. In line with

what I am saying, it is amazing to note
the number of community psychology programs
that have grown up at the master's level--
all of this in the face of no real definition of community psychology, no jobs in
the field for community psychologists, and
no agreed-upon training programs at the
Ph.D. level.

THE CAMPUS COMMUNITY
MENTAL HEALTH CENTER

About five years ago I had the opportunity to study the campus community
mental health center. In 1966 I obtained
a grant from the National Institute of
Mental Health for a program entitled "Graduate Training in Community Mental Health."
This was one of the first programs with
an arts and science base in the United
States. It was and is a modest program
with only six stipends. I was impressed
then, as I am now, with the complexities
of training in mental health. You will
note that I am saying mental health rather than community psychology. I don't
think that in 1967 it would have been possible to sell the term "community psychology" to many psychology departments. It
was just too new and the burgeoning community mental health movement demanded too
much investment to pay much attention to
community psychology. There were no internships for community mental health
oriented psychologists and so we had to
make some compromises within existing community mental health structures. Most of
the internships were pretty traditional
and this is understandable. Nobody had
much confidence or much experience in some

of the methods that are now pretty much
taken for granted. In 1968 I was offered
a challenge. I had complained bitterly
about the woeful state of mental health
services on the University of Texas campus. The President of the University ap-
pointed a committee to study ways of improving these services and this committee
met in May, 1968. In August, 1968, we
had the Whitman incident where Charles
Whitman climbed to the tower of the University of Texas campus and killed some
14 people and wounded about 25 more. Suddenly I became a prophet with some honor
in his own house, so to speak. I was offered the directorship of the Counseling
Center at University of Texas. This was
a place of good reputation with, of course,
a traditional counseling and guidance orientation. I looked upon the directorship
as a possibility for trying out some of
my ideas on campus-community mental health.
The President of the University, Norman
Hackerman, was and is an outstanding human being despite his tough exterior. I
accepted the challenge and in making me
Director he told me to go after quality
services and that he would back me all the
way. He never failed and I was able to
slowly begin putting into operation some
of my notions regarding mental health services.

You will recall that I knew nothing
about counseling. I wasn't trained in it.
And I set about recruiting people who had
a variety of ideas and who were dedicated
to trying out new techniques in the delivery of services. Jurisdictional boundaries tend to become obscured in this
type of undertaking. The basic strategy

is to consider the entire campus as a
series of resources and indeed the entire
community surrounding the campus as potential or actual resources. The strategy is "what is the best resource for the
problem presented by the student?" If
resources are lacking then the problem
is to construct them. Our crisis orientation is one in which the basic strategy
is "to get the students off the ropes and
into the center of the ring." Life itself
is the best therapist and the task is to
find out what works and doesn't work and
not to get stampeded into a variety of
perhaps popular but ineffective actions.
New types of manpower have to be developed
and we certainly did do this. We ran
housewives through a two-year half-time
program. They are all still working with
us. They've raised their kids, they love
their work, they're solid people. For
example, the best thing for a freshman in
crisis, girls in particular, is an understanding person to listen to her, not necessarily an up-tight graduate student.
The paraprofessionals are extremely well
adapted. They get down to business and,
more importantly, they know their business.

We set up probably the first 24-hour
telephone counseling program in the nation
and it's still going. We trained gradu-
ates and undergraduates in this service.
We also put in a lot of other things not
really germane to community psychology
per se.

One thing you learn in a campus community mental health approach, or for that
matter community psychology, is that you

have to be constantly evaluating. If you
simply set yourself up to render service,
eventually the service engulfs you and you
die. You have to take advantage of the
other resources on campus and off campus.
And you have to also begin to phase out
certain services that are not being as effective as you like. Perhaps the greatest challenge of all is the institution
of preventive service. We have a saying
on our campus that "He got his Ph.D. and
a divorce in the same month." I'm referring, of course, to the large number of
family breakups in graduate school. If
you ask a university for another $15,000
for a marital counselor, you're almost
sure to get it. If you ask for $5,000
for a preventive program, you're sure not
to get it. A strange thing! We pay much
attention to suicides and virtually no
attention to the infinitely greater number of living suicides on any campus or
any community. It's also strange, for
example, how little we really know about
the resources on our campus and I'll bet
that 50 percent of you listening to this
lecture don't even know half of the resources in your own university that could
be used or at least developed. One of the
paradoxes in the delivery of services is
that if you do a real good job, you become
very popular. Consequently, you become
innundated. How then can you still do a
good job and render quality mental health
services? Obviously you need a variety
of strategies--and one, of course, is preventive intervention. This means, for
example, finding ways in which to have an
on-going education program for the wives
of graduate students. It means also team-
ing up with financial aids to have a fi-

nancial counseling service close to the
married students' housing. It means
health lectures and day care centers
available to the married students. It
also means anticipatory guidance to the
extent of getting through to couples just
entering graduate school and pointing out
some of the hazards that are faced and
some of the constructive coping that can
take place. In so doing, one must not
lose sight of the resources in the community. For example, the campus ministry
have proven invaluable as marital counselors and educators. Their value has
increased by offering them consultation
and chances to upgrade their own skills.
If, as another example, there is need for
a detoxification unit in the community,
it might be well for the university to
assist the community in setting this up.
Detox units may be too expensive for the
university itself to establish. Moreover,
if you develop a university detox unit,
that means that the feds and the narcs
will be hassling you. The best way is to
spend some time negotiating with various
departments such as local and county police or the sheriff, and then find something that's worth it for them. For example, the county sheriff can be approached by telling him that if he has a detox
unit he need not have that many drunks in
the county jail over the weekend. He gets
terribly interested in a detox unit. If
you know your community, you know that 50
percent of the arrests are for alcohol,
especially on the weekend. Naturally a
county sheriff would be happy if "you'll
take all those lousy drunks off my hands."
A detox unit has other potential support-
ers. Big shots in the community who may

get arrested for drunken driving are better off taken to a detox unit rather than
to the county jail. That's how to apply
community psychology. One of the things
that I have found is that many of the
students do not really wish to understand
the resources, and come up with such simplistic ideas as cursing the city council
or insisting that the county commissioner
or the school board are a pack of conservative idiots. The reality of a community
psychology and community mental health
approach is simply that you have got to
learn how to work with the bad guys. It's
easy to succeed with the good boys, but
that's not the way the book is written.
Eventually you learn that even the bad
guys have got some needs with which you
may be able to help them. If you really
learn the system of the school and what
pressures the commissioners are under,
what sacrifices they make in terms of
time, then you are in a better position
to understand the psychology of the community. Another thing is quite important. You also have to give something to
these people. It's important, therefore,
for students to attend meetings of the
city council, the school board, and the
county commissioners. If it's politics,
so be it. From these emerge sophisticated
students and not enthusiastic amateurs.
It is only in this way that they can learn
that people on human services boards are
also human beings and they too are beset
by fantastic pressures and the need to
come up with answers on a rather immediate basis. I am proud of the fact that
the school superintendent of Austin saw
fit to consult with a number of top-level
psychologists about the problems of inte-

gration and to listen to some of their
suggestions. This was, of course, a good
model for the community psychology students to observe.

Good training in community psychology involves letting students roam out of
the Psychology Department and take full
advantage of the university in the best
sense of the word. If we are going to
emphasize management systems, then it is
better to have this from the department
of management. If you are going to have
students get some knowledge of community
organization in a more traditional sense,
then perhaps the School of Social Work or
Sociology is the place to go. Our own
program has benefited enormously from having students take, for example, the Sociology of Mental Health Services taught by
Ivan Belknap, who some of the older faculty may remember as being a pioneer in the
field by virtue of his publication of Human Problems of a State Mental Hospital
(1956). One of the most useful courses
that our community psychology students
take is a course in the College of Architecture on Urban Design. It is taught by
Raynell Parkins, a Black professor of
architecture who has also had enormous
experience in community organization.
Raynell really socks it to the students
and tries to impart to them the responsibility that architects should have for
betterment of the human condition and the
penalties they should pay for designs that
contribute to human misery.

I want to point out that the "super-
market" approach, where a large variety
of services is offered, teaches you that

certain things work for a period of time
and they they become less effective. For
example, a few years ago, about 1968, we
recognized that there was a need for an
all-night problem center. We called it
the Listening Ear and actually it was a
way to deal with a variety of problems
off campus. It was housed in the Metho-
dist Student Center and nominally they
were running it. We paid for the coordinator, the electricity, the telephone,
and did the training of the volunteers.
Gradually our evaluation indicated that
the students were moving out of the neighborhood away from campus and that other
resources were being opened for the students. The drug scene by about 1971 was
abating in Austin and the Listening Ear
was not being used that much. The Jesus
freaks, for example, had opened up the
Well, and the Middle Earth had been opened up as a crash pad for bad trips. We
abandoned the Listening Ear and went on
to help other organizations get started
such as Hotline and Switchboard, the latter designed to give information about
where people could stay for the night and
avail themselves of other resources within the town or university. The important
factor here too is to have the student
involved both in the delivery of service
and in evaluation.

One of the lessons one learns in
community psychology is that interventions and resources are in constant need
of reassessment, change, and perhaps out-
right abolition. Sometimes a very much
needed resource cannot function because
the community is not facing up to the re-
sponsibility--this is especially true when

information about the family life of the
middle class or power structure may become more public. About 1968, for example, our graduate students recognized
the need for services to teenagers who
were "on the lam" or running away from
home. They were influenced by the work
in Haight-Ashbury and the book about Huckleberry House, a haven for runaways in
the Haight-Ashbury district. The graduate
students obtained the cooperation of a local church and quickly organized and equip-
ped a rather impressive set-up. All the
work was contributed by volunteers except
our program put in money for a half-time
coordinator. It was frankly a way to get
the graduate students some "action" feeling, as they were contained by a clinical
program that was rather traditional. (At
that time community psychology was part
of a clinical program. It emerged as an
independent program only in 1972.) My
own experience forewarned of great difficulties in the community but frankly, I
wanted the students to learn on their own
and they certainly did. They learned,
for example, that there were an enormous
number of youngsters under 18 who were
on the move away from home. In winter,
there was a migration from the north towards the south. They also learned that
not everyone fleeing from home has been
hassled by unreasonable parents. They
learned that some youngsters are extremely disturbed, some are untrustworthy, and
others are frankly in it for the adventure
and their own game. Learning about a mixed bag rather than a pure article is a
very important step. The organization
was called the Raft and it was, of course,
named after the raft in Huckleberry Finn.

The students had a great time but it soon
became clear that the Raft was a threat
to the community. Why? Too many children
of prominent families in the city were
running away and taking sanctuary in the
Raft. The powers that be moved against
the Raft as a "destroyer of family relations" and there was the usual harassment
by narcs, etc. The graduate students
tried their best to keep runaways from
bringing any type of drugs into the Raft
and they by far and large succeeded. They
maintained proper decorum and all males
and females were appropriately chaperoned.
They made efforts to get families together.
The Raft finally had to give up because
the funds were drying up based on withdrawal of community support in terms of
donations. Nevertheless, the need per-
sisted and, of course, still persists today. In recognition of this, a number
of other resources and sanctuaries have
sprung up away from the campus and perhaps
more focused on children of lower socioeconomic classes. When they get into
trouble the community is not that much
threatened and if they "spill the beans"
about their family life, it is not very
embarrassing to the powers that be. What
I want to emphasize, again, is that any
beneficial force in the community will
also have negative aspects. A sophisticated community psychologist recognizes
these negative aspects and attempts to
deal with them before they become too
strong and overwhelm the organization itself.

RESEARCH

Quite naturally a university professor must do some research. I have done a little myself but for the last two years I have been too busy developing various organizations to do much. I am interested in the fate of transfer students who come to the University of Texas and the types of services that can be given them to facilitate their succeeding in a high quality state-supported school. On a more preventive level, I am interested in the whole area of married students, as I noted earlier. Hiring a marriage counselor is something that administrators understand. However, a preventive educational approach is more difficult to find. From a community psychology point of view, the approach I would advocate is one in which some of the causes of the break-up are studied. Some of these are quite easily identified, such as: (1) the rapidly widening educational gap between the male graduate student and the wife/worker; (2) the value gap that quickly develops; and (3) the mistaken belief that once he gets his masters or Ph.D. or other degree, all the problems will vanish and the world will be rosy. Obviously, some anticipatory guidance and rapid intervention techniques are needed. The problem is how to employ them and how to intervene in a student housing set-up. The set-up is predominantly "management" oriented and just beginning to understand prevention. It is my hope that we can have a married-student housing special services which will include courses in adult education given in the evenings, and discussion groups and other methods focusing directly on the problems

of the young marrieds including financial
planning resources, child care, and the
like. The basic purpose is to reduce the
communication gap that inevitably develops when one of the partners is going to
school. There is an aspect of male chau-
vinism in all this because I am presuming
the man is going to school. It might very
well be the other way around and the man
would be working and the woman going to
school. No matter, it is a question of
human relations and intervention rather
than picking up the casualties of a social system.

Another problem area similar to this
one is that of high-rise dormitories and
how to make them more attractive to students. Here there is an incentive for
the university, unlike in housing for married students. The reason for the incentive is that the university is in danger
of not having the dormitories full. This
is a problem all over the United States
and one for which management-oriented ad-
ministrations now have to look more carefully at spending money for programs to
make dormitories more attractive. Of
course, had the universities bothered to
involve some of the students in the planning of dormitories or in the programs a
while ago, the might not now be in such
a pickle. As a matter of fact, it is
doubtful whether they would have constructed high-rise dormitories at all. I would
predict that eventually dormitories will
be changed in terms of eased restrictions
and various alternatives offered to students so that they become more attractive
as living places. However, I also predict
that campuses will no longer be virtually

self-contained; higher percentages of
students will live off campus. Already
it appears that the two-bedroom apartment
is the most desirable type of living arrangement for students, that is, from the
student's point of view.

I am also quite concerned about a
significant proportion of our population
that presently exists on public welfare.
If welfare is a reality, then cannot people exist more effectively as human beings while on welfare? What's the matter
with them acquiring competence in sports,
liking the arts, in developing taste for
classical music, gourmet cooking, and
wine tasting? One of the problems is that
they are on welfare and they are not supposed to be happy. We get upset with people who are happy while living on other
people's money so to speak. On the other
hand, living on other people's money is
to some extent part and parcel of the
American system.

What I am asking for is the possibility of some careful study in which we
find ways in which people can live on welfare but also live a fuller life. More
to the point, I would be interested in
how people can get off welfare. Suppose
we took certain families and gave them
increased monthly allotments until we
found the combination of factors that allowed them to get off welfare and reduce
dependency. We would ask such questions
as: At what point is there reached a
critical mass or obstacle? It seems obvious that in the big cities the obstacle
is the cost of rent. As people start to
move upward they get zapped with huge

housing costs and they are stuck. I would
like to study how much extra it takes to
get a family on welfare to take more risk
behavior so that they might be able to
subsist on their own. Or if the reality
of a subsidized population remains, what
are the benefits of having a well-subsi-
dized population rather than one at a sub-
sistence subsidy level?

I am also interested in how universities work. It is amazing how complex
they are and how little they have been
studied. I am very pessimistic about the
survival of the great state-supported universities. I do not think they will be
able to continue, simply because they have
failed to make use of their internal resources and they are turning quickly from
a leadership to a management orientation.
In this regard, they resemble the decline
of the great cities where the cities are
now "used" by persons in the suburbs.
These same persons do not identify with
the city and are little concerned with
its internal problems.

I could go on telling you about some
of these research areas but I would prefer
to head towards a conclusion of my presentation by some speculation as to where
we are going in the area of community
psychology. I have tried to give you some
idea of how I got into the thing and, as
you may have gathered, sometimes I would
like to get out of the area. These are
not times for great optimism, yet one must
have some sort of faith that man and his
adaptive ability will be able to come
through these difficult times. Community
psychology is different from community

mental health and different from clinical psychology. This is so even though
presently there are no positions labelled "community psychologist."

What of the future? I hope that in
five years or so we have a different community psychology than we have now. I
hope that we will direct more attention
to social systems intervention methods
and planning than presently exists. We
have not held a Boulder Conference on
training in community psychology because
some of us have not wanted to crystallize
the area. Clinical did this at Boulder
and has paid the penalty ever since. I
see new models coming down the road and
I urge that we experiment with the new
ones. Students who are interested in
exactitude and cannot stand ambiguity
and lack of structure should definitely
not, repeat not, get into the area of
community psychology. They should recognize that this is an area in tremendous
and rapid transition and if they are looking for models and structure they are in
the wrong field. One of our great tasks
at present is to avoid the tendency toward
"neatness" that some of our academic colleagues place upon us. The most important problems of human beings do not lend
themselves to neat models. The day may
come when this may be so but that day is
not yet here. The only model I employ
for community psychology is a threefold
one: (1) where is the money coming from;
(2) who are the professionals involved
and what are their intramural and extra-
mural battles; and (3) who are the consumers of the products of community psychology and how do the consumers feed back

into the system? This is a simple model,
yet one that is not even faced in teaching in graduate schools. The sources of
funding and the professional relationships between professionals and the tar-
get populations all have to be studied
separately and simultaneously. I would
urge, therefore, that community psychology programs let their students begin
to understand the forces of funding and
the functions of other professionals besides psychologists. I would urge also
that psychologists really begin to understand communities not in a detached sense
but via a living everyday approach. The
orientation that I would urge would be
on how communities meet crisis--what are
their resources and what are their reper-
toires of coping responses. Along this
line, it will be interesting for students
to see whether the prestigious universities in the United States will be able to
survive in community psychology terms.
They, too, are going through what may be
referred to as a "transformational crisis." They became prestigious universities by pure research and dedication to
a course of action that paid off in the
past. Will it pay off in the future? I
am not sure. I am sure, however, that the
"hungrier" universities may put together
packages of great attraction to students
and scholars and that they may be the
ones to carry on cooperative ventures
with communities. All this remains to
be seen in the future.

One last word about research. I feel
that in many ways the rebellion against
traditional psychology has tended to de-
nigrate research and evaluation. I want

to make the statement that careful, hon-
est evaluation and good research are ab-
solutely essential for developing community psychology. In fact, a whole new
body of knowledge will have to be generated and this will require new methods.
I deplore the fact that research is sometimes attacked by applied psychologists.
I deplore the fact that some community
psychologists tend to be a little nihi-
listic with regard to research. On the
contrary, community psychology will have
to produce a new breed of cat so to speak
--a person knowledgeable in quasi-experimental designs, multivariant analysis,
and decision-making theory along with his
knowledge of the community. This is a
tall order but an order that we must in
some way partially fulfill if we are to
generate the knowledge that will be needed for a viable community psychology of
the future.

For those of you who contemplate a
career in the araa of community psychology, I counsel courage and patience.
This is a new area that has sprung up in
response to concerns of many human beings. I predict undergraduate majors in
the broad areas of community psychology
and I predict, eventually, a change in
function so that the community psychologist will more likely be a person at the
master's level functioning in various
roles and settings in the community while
community psychology in terms of its research and its conceptual basis will re-
side in universities and professional
schools. The theory and practice of community psychology must, like all other
disciplines, undergo constant reconsider-

ation and constant enrichment from the feedback from community settings. Thank you.

REFERENCES

Belknap, I. Human problems of a state mental hospital. New York: McGraw-Hill, 1956.

Bloom, B. Training the psychologist for a role in community change. Division of Community Psychology Newsletter, 3, (#3)--Special Issues, November, 1969.

Campbell, D. T., and Stanley, J. C. Experimental and quasi-experimental designs for research. Chicago: Rand McNally, 1963.

Joint Commission on Mental Illness and Health. Action for mental health. New York: Basic Books, 1961.

Miller, K. S., and Iscoe, I. The concept of crisis. Human Organization, 1963, 22, 195-201.

Warren, R. L. Mental health planning and Model Cities: "Hamlet or hellzapoppin." Community Mental Health Journal, 1971, 7, 39-49.

INDEX

Academic psychology:
    and community psychology, 164, 171
    function of, 170
    and methodology, 171
    research in, 170-171
Albee, G. W., 53
Allen, G. J., 62, 66, 67, 68, 77
Allen, G. W., 66
Allport, F., 14, 15
American Journal of Community Psychology, 3
American Psychological Association:
    Boulder Conference, 123, 219
    Division of Community Psychology, 3, 89, 163, 175
Ames, A., 14, 15
Anderson, L. S., 3
Ansama, J. W., 49
Architecture:
    of community mental health centers, 108-109
    and community organization, 211
Argyris, C., 165
Aronson, C. F., 61
Assessment:
    ecology of, 158-161
    of environment. See Environment
    of settings. See Settings

Bambrough, B., 49
Bard, M., 163
Barker, R., 149
Bauer, R., 20
Behavior modification, 42, 67, 71
    in ward environment, 62-63
Behrens, W. W., 23
Belknap, I., 211
Bennett, C. C., 3, 14, 87
Bentley, A. F., 15, 16, 17
Betz, B. J., 48
Boston Conference, 1-4, 14, 86-90
    emphases of, 9-10
    planning of, 87-88
Boston University, 83, 87
    Human Relations Laboratory, 87
Boulder Conference, 123, 219
Brown, M., 88
Caine, E., 77
California, University of at Los Angeles,
    182
Campus community mental health, 205-214
    need for marital counseling in, 208-
        209
Cantril, H., 14, 15
Caplan, G., 29, 85
Carew, M., 131
Carkhuff, R. R., 48
Causality, three-way view of, 16
Center for Community Studies, George Pea-
    body College, 26-27
Change agentry, 6, 35, 41-42, 113-114
Chinsky, J., 5, 6, 7, 41-82
Classroom environment, 140-141
    scale, 136-141
Clinical psychologist, limitations of
    role, 85
Clinical psychology:
    Boulder model of, 219
    and community mental health, 1
    and community psychology, 163, 202

limitations of, 41-44
training in, 53, 124-125
Coleman, J., 24
Collaborative intervention design, 7, 50-53, 61
College students. See undergraduates
Community:
        assessing needs of, 98-103, 156
        as a dynamic organization, 22-23
        education of, 103
        organization, 211
        philosophical issues of, 20-21
        psychologists' relationships with, 33-34
        quality of life in, 25-36
        resources in, 210-211
        and social planning, 98-103
        and stress, 116
        theory of, 21-23
Community events, monitoring of, 6
Community groups, working with, 54
Community mental health:
        administration. See Mental health administration
        in campus setting, 206-214
        and community psychology, 14, 88, 164-165, 205-206, 218-219
        need for community support in, 214
        origin of, 1
        training in, 88, 90-91, 205
Community mental health centers, architectural design of, 108-109
Community Mental Health Centers Act, 13-14, 105
Community Mental Health Journal, 3, 89
Community organization, 89
Community programs:
        assessment techniques and, 61
        community input into, 101-103
        coordination of, 109-110
        essential services of, 103

establishment of, 100-103
funding of, 111
implementation and evaluation of, 49-
    73
institutionalization of, 54-55
personal relationships and, 57
and planning for mental health, 110-
    111
related to mood, 28
resources in social systems, 57-58
selection of personnel for, 55-56
special features of, 53-58
Community psychologist:
becoming a, 181-222
changing roles of, 221
as consultant, 51
education of, 123-179
functions of, 219
lifestyle of, 168-169
professional accountability of, 168
training of, 87, 89, 202
university as a setting for, 8, 53-54
Community psychology, 123
and academic psychology, 164, 171
accountability, 164
case study approach in, 166-167
and clinical psychology, 163, 172-173,
    202
and community mental health, 14, 88,
    164-165, 205-206, 218-219
competence in, 164
concerns of, 20-21
as content area, 162-169
contributions to, 72-73
defined, 2
and ecological analysis, 151
ecological ideology of, 23
energy perspective and, 23-26
entry into, 83-90, 181-193
focus for, 127
future of, 36, 73-77, 174-176, 218-

222
and mental health administration,
        83-122
model for, 219-220
need for evaluation in, 75, 220-221
need for methodological tradition,
        166-168, 174
origin of, 1-3, 18-21
philosophy and, 21-22
research in, 26-34, 172, 215-222
research models of, 34-35
research training in, 73, 204-205
and the rest of psychology, 14-15
resources for, 148-149
roots in psychology, 14-18
roots in social psychology and social
        change, 18-21
and technology, 6, 23-26
theories of change, 151
training, funding of, 75-76
training in, 3, 8, 42, 50, 72, 90-91,
        173, 210-211
university as a setting for, 156-176,
        203-205
view backward and forward, 13-40
Connecticut, University of, 6, 47, 50, 58,
        77
Consultant, 105
Continuing education, 24
Cooper, L., 142
Cooper, S., 3, 87
Corcoran, C. A., 66
Counseling Center at University of Texas,
        206-214
Counseling center, staffing of, 206-207
Cowen, E., 6, 44, 45, 50, 63, 77, 163
Crisis intervention, 102
        and campus community mental health,
                212
        in counseling center, 207
Crisis theory, 29

Dailey, W., 62, 66
D'Augelli, A. R., 49
Deinstitutionalization, 114
Denzin, N., 18
Detoxification Units, 209
Deviance, 6
Dewey, J., 15, 16, 17
Dittman, A. T., 127
Dizurrilla, T. J., 70
Dormitories, future of, 216-217
Drugs, as social controls, 46
Duke University, 85-86
Ecological analogy, 8, 125, 135, 143-151,
     158
     application of, 151-156
     and assessment, 158-161
     defined, 144
     principles of, 144-156
     in schools, 152
Ecology, 3, 16-18, 89
     of assessment, 158-161
     and mental health, 88
Economics, 89
Education, 23-25
     preschool, 58-61. See also Schools
Elementary school:
     behavior modification in, 71
     companionship program in, 70
Endler, N. S., 127-133
Environments:
     assessment of, 165
     and ecological perspective, 135-136
Epidemiology, 89
Etzioni, A., 24
Evaluation:
     of mental health programs, 117-118
     need for in community psychology,
          220-221
Fairweather, G. W., 76
Forrester, J., 31
General systems theory, 17

George Peabody College, 6, 26
Gestalt theory, 17
Glidewell, J., 87
Golann, S., 13, 44, 175
Goldenberg, I., 163
Goldfried, M. R., 70
Goodman, G., 48
Gordon, T., 20
Group Assessment of Interpersonal Traits,
      48
Hackerman, N., 206
Harris, J., 62
Harris, T. A., 20
Harvard School of Public Health, 85, 86,
      125
Hassol, L., 3
Headstart, 58
Helsing, K. J., 30
Highbee, K. L., 125
Hirschowitz, R. G., 120, 121
Hofstadter, R., 19
Housing, 60
Human services, directory of, 107
Hunt, J., 127, 133
Illich, I., 24
Inservice training, 67
Institutionalization:
      of community programs, 54-55
      effect on behavior of, 67
Institutional standards, compliance with,
      114-115
Interactions, person-setting, 126, 127-135
Interaction recording system, 64-68
Intervention:
      and institutional affiliation, 161-162
      planning for, 160
      preventive, 208-209
      research in designing, 169
      theories of, 165
Iscoe, I., 5, 8, 9, 163, 181-222
Journal of Community Psychology, 3

Journal of Personality and Social Psycho-
      logy, 125
Kahn, R., 150
Kantor, J. R., 17
Katz, D., 150
Kaufman, B., 136
Kelly, G., 124
Kelly, J., 8, 55, 71, 88, 125, 143, 163,
      168
Kiesler, D. J., 47
Klaber, M. M., 63
Klein, D. C., 3, 87
Kleopfer, B., 182
Korner, I., 88
Larcen, S., 69
Law enforcement, 89
Lawson, R., 124
Levin, H., 19, 21
Lewin, K., 15
Lippitt, R., 20, 35
Lochman, J. E., 71
Long, N., 22
Mann, P., 163
Married students, preventive intervention
      for, 215-216
Maryland, University of, 142
Massachusetts Department of Mental Health,
      7, 83, 91-98
Massachusetts Psychological Association,
      94
Massachusetts, University of, 4, 181
Mead, G. H., 16
Meadows, D. H., 23
Meadows, D. L., 23
Mental health, lobbying for, 107-108
Mental health administration, 91-121
      and community psychology, 83-122
      future of, 118-120
      and primary prevention, 115-117
      and social change, 93-94
Mental Health Administrator:

Nassol, L., 87
National Institute of Mental Health, Mental Health Study Center, 6
Newbrough, J. R., 5, 13-40
Nisbet, R., 173, 174
Nixon, Richard M., 19, 105
Nonprofessionals, 53, 54, 120
    indigenous, 88
    as prevention agents, 58-59
    selection of, 48
    therapeutic attributes of, 47-49
Ochberg, F. M., 146, 152
Ohio State University, 8, 123, 124, 125
Papanek, V., 25
Paraprofessionals, 120, 148
    training of, 207
    See also Nonprofessionals
Parkins, R., 211
Pearl, A., 88
Personality, 147
Person-setting interactions. See Inter-
    actions
Pervin, L., 130
Pierce, W. D., 141
Poser, E. G., 44
Preschool education program, 58-61
Primary prevention:
    defined, 99n
    in elementary school, 69-70
    and mental health administration,
        115-117
    programs, 74
Privacy, protection of, 33-34
Psychologists:
    changing status of, 91-96
    training of, 25
Psychotherapy, function of, 203
Public health, 89
    model, 14
Racial tension, in schools, 152
Randers, J., 23

Rappaport, J., 6, 44, 45, 46, 50, 63, 77
Raush, H. L., 127, 133, 166
Rawls, S., 20
Reiff, R., 21, 88
Revel, J. F., 20
Research:
    in designing interventions, 169
    ecological validity of, 130
    need for methodology in community
        psychology, 166-168
    models of, 18, 34-35, 124
    schools as settings for, 129-135
    systems level, 73
    traditional methodology, 166
    training in community psychology, 73,
        204-205
Resources:
    assessment of, 148-149, 159-161
    cycling of, 155-156
    in schools, 159-161
Retardates, ward behavior of, 62-68
Rhodes, W. C., 26
Rochester State Hospital, 43, 63
Rochester State Hospital Project, 44-47
Rochester, University of, 6, 44, 50
Rosenblum, G., 3, 5, 7, 83-122
Rotter, J., 51, 53, 77
Royce, R. B., 15
Ryan, W., 74
Sanford, N., 14
Sarason, S., 163, 165
Schindler-Rainman, E., 20, 35
Schneider, B., 142
Schofield, W., 44
Schools:
    assessment of change in, 141-143
    assessment of settings in, 141-143
    case study approach in, 152
    classroom environment, 140-141
    consultation in, 134, 157-161
    elementary, 69-70, 71, 158

functions of, 131-132
goals of, 150
intervention in, 158
multilevel intervention in, 68-72
organizational structure of, 150
policy making in, 144-146
primary prevention in, 116-117
racial tension in, 152
referrals in, 159
as research settings, 129-141, 143
resources in, 159-161
satisfaction with, 132, 134
and social change, 150
Scientist-professional model, 123
Scribner, S., 4
Secondary prevention, 129
defined, 99n
Seeman, J., 26
Selinger, H. V., 70
Sensitivity groups, selection procedures
for, 49
Settings:
assessment of, 8, 126, 128, 147, 151,
158-159
creation of, 165
Smith, W., 30
Social change, 19-21, 76-77
and schools, 150
mental health administrator and, 93-
94
Social planning, 156
Social problems:
research on, 53
and social activism, 41-42
Social systems intervention, 219
Society, voluntary, 35
South Shore Mental Health Center, 7, 84,
86, 87, 90, 102, 116
Spencer, F. W., 66
Spiesman, J., 87
Stanford University Medical Center, 126,

156
Stern, G., 136
Stress, 32
Student power movement, 152-156
Students:
    graduate, as supervisors, 50-51
    as therapeutic agents, 44-49, 50-53
    See also undergraduates
Supervision, training in, 51
Swampscott Conference. See Boston Confer-
    ence
Systematic research, social change and, 76
Systems modelling, 31
Taylor, T. T., 127
Telephone counseling, 207
Tennessee Valley Authority, 25
Tertiary prevention, 129
    defined, 99n
Texas, University of, 9, 206
Thaw, J., 62
Thomas, P. H., 61
Todd, D. M., 143, 157
Transactional functionalism, 14, 15-16
Transactionalism, origin of, 17
Treatment, priorities for, 115
Trickett, E. J., 5, 8, 123-179
Truax, C. B., 82
Tutor-companions, 59-61
Undergraduates, 52, 54, 72
    as therapeutic agents, 45, 50, 52
    as tutor-companions, selection of, 59
    See also Students
Universities:
    survival of, 218
    and community psychology, 156-176,
        203-214
    functions, of, 170
Urban planning, 89
Veit, S., 62, 64, 66, 67
von Bertalanffy, L., 17
Ward environment:

        assessment of, 62-68
        and staff/patient ratios, 66
Ward interactions, observation of, 63-68
Washington University, 87
Webb, E. J., 18
Weber, M., 21
Welfare, function of, 217-218
Wells, M. G., 125
Wheeler, H., 20
Whitehorn, J. C., 48
Whitman, C., 206
Witmer, L., 1
Woodworth, 14
Yale University, 8
        Psycho-Educational Clinic, 8, 156-157